Cooking to Please Finicky Kids

Cooking to Please Finicky Kids

By BETTY WASON

ASSOCIATION PRESS
published with
FRED KERNER/PUBLISHING PROJECTS
New York

Association Press, 291 Broadway, New York 10007

SBN: 8096-1718-8

Library of Congress catalog card number: 69-18839

72

Printed in the United States of America

CONTENTS

Part I

Part II

PART I

THE SITUATION

Mealtime, say all the psychologists and child experts, should be a happy time, an occasion when the family joyously breaks bread together.

Then mealtime arrives, your little cherubs are called to the table, and what happens?

"What's that stuff?" asks Johnny. "I don't want any."

"Don't give me any, either," echoes little sister.

"Carrots again?" protests their elder brother. "Jeez, we're *always* having carrots."

What's a loving mother supposed to do? When the plates are pushed away still piled with food, should she scream, "You will eat every morsel on that plate before you can leave the table!"

Or plead, "But dear, it's *delicious!* See, Mommy and Daddy are eating all of theirs."

Or weep, "Johnny, what's *wrong* with you? Why don't you have any appetite?"

Or pay no attention at all?

The experts always advise paying no attention. I wonder how many of them have raised finicky eaters themselves?

There are no hard and fast rules for getting children to eat properly. What works with one child will fail dismally with another. It's some consolation to keep reminding yourself that little Johnny will not starve even if for three meals in a row he eats no more than a single spoonful of mashed potatoes. There isn't a case on record of a finicky child who has died of starvation.

The trouble is, there are plenty of finicky children suffering from malnutrition. It's all very well to say one should simply ignore a child's lack of mealtime appetite. Half an hour after the table has been cleared, chances are you will find him munching potato chips, or finishing a bottle of pop, or licking the crumbs from the cake plate.

And what can you do to stop such snacking? Put padlocks on the pantry doors and the refrigerator?

Say the experts, "Let them alone. Natural selectivity will make children turn to the foods they need when the time comes."

Such a theory sounds like good sense and in the old days, before snacks were so overly available, it may have worked. The trouble today is that keeping a child from snacking between meals is all but impossible—unless he is kept in solitary confinement. The kids beat a path to the door of the neighbor's house where the supply of soft drinks is always plentiful, or they are treated to lollipops by an indulgent storekeeper, or they put their pennies in the slot machine at the supermarket and fill their pockets with sour balls.

Some between-meal snacking is inevitable. If it's kept under control, it may do no harm. But how do you keep it under control?

My finicky child has now become a teen-ager. She is in robust health, and she still eats like a canary. Her school-day breakfasts are woefully inadequate, according to everything I, as a home economist, have been taught. Frankly, I worry over how little she eats at dinner. But she thrives. The doctor assures me she's as "healthy as a young horse."

The conscientious parent simply has to play this problem by ear. Sometimes it is necessary to insist that certain foods be eaten before the child may leave the table. On occasion one must plead, "But take at least one bite of this—really, it's delicious!" And again there are times when punishment is necessary, when a youngster has gorged on forbidden snacks just before a meal. Finding the route between nagging and common sense is the parental problem, and it's never a straight path.

GENERAL GUIDELINES

Three things must never be forgotten.

First, since your child obviously does not have a robust appetite, don't expect him (or her) to eat much. **Second,** make food at mealtime as appealing as possible. And **third,** *try* not to fuss about it.

The last is the hardest of all. When you have gone to the trouble of preparing a meal, whether for one other person or six, you like your efforts to be appreciated. The sight of food left upon a plate is a kind of snub. Or so you feel.

Your reaction is psychological. So is *his*. The more you insist he must eat more, the less he wants—and the more worry. And in just no time at all, *not eating* becomes his way of getting extra attention.

Often there are other factors involved, too. But, for the moment, let's assume it's as simple as this. How do you reconcile yourself to this bird-like appetite? How do you handle this exasperating situation? Here are some suggestions:

Put tiny, tiny portions on his plate. If they are so small, he wants more, *then* you can express pleasure in his having such a good appetite today. (From now on "he" may be interpreted as "or she." Don't think we're ignoring the girls. Their appetites, if anything, tend to be even skimpier than the boys'.)

Don't force foods on him you know he dislikes. So he doesn't like spinach! Let him get his roughage by eating an apple or carrot sticks.

(As a young child, my daughter always preferred raw vegetables to cooked. Now as a teen-ager she likes both, and amazes me by being a better vegetable- than meat-eater. I can't promise it will work this way for your finicky ones; they may rebel against raw vegetables and fruits as vehemently as the cooked ones—but it's worth a try. *Anything* is worth a try.)

It is never wise to cook a different vegetable, or a different meat, just because the one being served to the rest of the family is on your finicky child's foods-I-most-dislike list. To go to this much trouble is making too much of a fuss about the whole thing.

Another method is to try putting an eyedropper-sized portion of the disliked food on his plate, simply because everyone else is getting some. But don't say one single word if it's still on his plate at the end of the meal. Of course, there's the danger that when you put that miniscule helping on his plate, he may let out a wild scream, "I *hate* spinach. Don't give me any of that stuff!" and push his plate to the middle of the table—or onto the floor. Very well. Don't give him any. Ignore him. Change the subject. The more violent his reaction, the more you can be sure this is all a put-up job, designed to get attention. Ask someone else at the table (not the screamer) how the ball game turned out, or whether they think it's a good day to go to the beach. If the plate is on the floor, let it stay there until the meal is finished—and make the screamer remain at his place at table.

(What is this doing to *your* nerves? Plenty! It's uphill for you all the way. But, courage! It will all turn out right in the end.)

Include favorite foods of his in the menu with reasonable frequency. Emphasis is on the word *reasonable.* Youngsters often develop passionate yearnings for one food and want it day after day after day. "You haven't had spaghetti for a *long* time," he will protest if three days have passed since spaghetti was last on the menu. At least, this is what may happen during the period when spaghetti is his obsession. Then one day, you will proudly announce, "We're having spaghetti for dinner tonight," and to your astonishment he will whine, "Spaghetti *again!* Why do we *always* have to have spaghetti?"

By this time the obsession has turned to French fries (or pizzas, or hot dogs, or maybe dill pickles!). So now every third day you will hear the complaint, "Why don't we ever have French fries any more?"

You can't hope to win with a finicky eater, no matter how hard you try.

Make food look good to eat. This doesn't mean garnishing the roast with carrot curls or radish roses. But it does mean presenting food attractively. Broiled or roast meats are more irresistible when crisply browned on the outside—without being burned. If the roast doesn't have that succulent look when the thermometer indicates it is almost done, baste with a little fat, or brush with just a little Kitchen Bouquet (or Gravymaster) diluted in water to give it a brown-glazed look. Take care in cooking vegetables to undercook them, so that they will be as bright in color as possible—and retain the most food value at the same time.

(When cooking spinach, broccoli or asparagus, leave the lid ajar so that steam may escape—for steam dulls the green color, and bright-colored vegetables seem actually to taste better than those that are limp and dull.)

When planning meals, remember to balance colors and textures. Avoid serving two white foods on the same plate (such as boiled potatoes and cauliflower), or two fried foods, or all soft-textured foods. With macaroni and cheese, for example, you might serve broccoli and broiled tomato slices. With pork chops, candied sweet potatoes and green peas. With barbecued spare ribs, yellow rice and lima beans.

Bring foods to table in attractive serving dishes. A bit of garnish often helps to make food look more tempting. If a pumice-colored stew tastes marvelous but looks deadly, brighten it with a bit of minced parsley sprinkled over the top just before serving. Sieved egg yolk or crumbled cooked bacon sprinkled over the top of split pea soup will make the soup look more appealing—and add nutrition, too. When mashed potatoes are piled in the serving dish, make a hollow in the center, place a lump of butter or margarine there so it will melt to a golden pool.

To the best of your ability, keep family mealtimes free from tension or argument. Within the intimacy of the family, all of us tend to spout off impulsively. We say what we feel, without giving a second thought to the effect on others. And that's the way it should be—within reason. But when talk becomes fretful, or argumentative, or controversial, it's time to call a halt. This applies to mother and dad even more than to the youngsters. If grown-ups can't provide an example of self-control, how can we expect the children to restrain themselves? If it's one of the children who is the worst offender, he must be asked to leave the table. If it's the man of the house, the little woman can only plead, "Please, dear, not before the children." But if it's the little woman herself who's to blame, heaven help her offspring.

Dessert should be served only to those who have

cleaned their plates (within reason). Some nutrition experts argue that denying dessert to children who have not finished the main course only serves to embellish the dessert with more importance than it deserves. Maybe so, but if a child does not have appetite enough to finish the meat-and-potatoes course, isn't it logical to conclude he hasn't appetite enough for strawberry shortcake or lemon meringue pie, either? The point should be made in the beginning, however, before the meal starts, as part of the happy announcement of the dessert that's waiting to appear. Often it's surprising to see how quickly the meat loaf is downed when it's known to be the first goal-post on the way to a devil's-food-cake finish.

But once a rule like this is established, you must be firm. If you give in just one time, your finicky eater will be sure he can twist your arm again in future. Children are geniuses when it comes to this kind of finagling.

And what about those desserts which are so nutritious your child really needs to have some—such as baked apples, milk-rich vanilla pudding, or good milk-and-egg cup custards? These will still be good later, either as between-meal snacks or for dessert following another meal. Johnny isn't going to starve.

Discipline is important. Calm-voiced, no-wavering, sensible discipline.

Keep only nutritious snacks on hand. There are some children whose appetite seems to disappear at mealtime, but between meals they become positively ravenous. Some nutritionists say let them eat between meals, as long as they are eating good-for-you foods. I have found just one flaw in this theory. The human animal is a creature of habit, and any child who establishes a 10 A.M. and 3 P.M. meal pattern instead of the family's noon and evening meal times (which is what the regular between-meal snacker is doing) is causing mother a great deal of unnecessary work and bother. On the other hand, a between-meal apple or carrot stick is a very good thing and allowing slices of hard-cooked egg on potato chips in late afternoon may be the only way you can get your finicky one to touch eggs at all.

The important thing is to see that your poor eater gets essential nutrition, and with the least possible fuss. If he is exposed only to good-for-you snack foods—and in this way eats what he should have at his own schedule—accept this as the best possible temporary solution and be happy.

More detailed suggestions will follow as to what such snacks might consist of, and recipes for nutritious snacks will be found in the recipe section.

IS LACK OF APPETITE CAUSE FOR ALARM?

Inevitably a conscientious parent will worry that poor appetite is a sign of poor health.

To allay your fears, do consult your family doctor—but not in the child's presence. The doctor probably will say he can only determine whether the poor appetite is cause for alarm by giving the child a thorough physical examination. In this case, tell your offspring that taking a physical is a routine thing—everyone needs such an examination yearly. (If your child is in school, very likely the school will request that he have such a general examination.) Whatever you do, don't let the child know it's his poor appetite that's the reason for the trip to the doctor, because most children *love* to go to the doctor's office. It makes them feel important. Such trips could make your youngster even more finicky than before.

Here are some possible causes of poor appetite. Consider each, one by one, to see whether one or more of them fits your case.

1) **Physical make-up.** Some individuals simply do not need as much food as others. There are wide differences in individual basic metabolism.

2) **Nervous tension.** We live in a nerve-wracking world and children are sensitive to the many pressures and fears that affect us all.

3) **Allergies.** These are sensitivities to certain foodstuffs (or to elements in the atmosphere). Often allergies are caused, or at least aggravated, by tension. My daughter, for example, has a sensitivity to milk; it causes her to have intense stomach cramps and diarrhea. Yet one summer when she went off to camp, after a specialist had advised that she should not consume milk in any form, she drank milk with all the other campers and wasn't bothered by it a bit. The open air life she was leading apparently cleared up the tensions that had affected her at home. I have since observed that it's on school days when milk upsets her most, and can only conclude that the tensions of school life are as much to blame as the latent sensitivity to the milk. Nevertheless, if allergies are upsetting your child's system and causing real physical anguish, you will have to adjust his diet accordingly, for this in turn will affect appetite.

4) **Desire for attention.** This doesn't mean your young one is simply a conniving brat. Maybe he really needs more attention. Perhaps you are so preoccupied with problems, or worries, or the relentless schedules of a modern mother's day, he feels neglected. But fussing over his lack of appetite is *not* the kind of attention he should have. Better to make it a story at bedtime, or a sharing of some fun experience, or frequent gestures of affection.

5) **Desire to leave the table to play.** He may have been involved in a game with neighbor children just before being called in for dinner, or your daughter may have become so engrossed in the dream world of her doll family, she resents being brought back to reality, or a budding artist may just have discovered the creative joy of finger paints or crayons on big blank sheets of paper. Or a television program may be much more interesting than sitting at table with grown-ups.

Many American parents today set their youngsters in front of the TV screen at mealtime, with TV dinners on TV tables. If the show is good, the children may down the warmed-over commercially prepared food without even knowing what they are eating. It's an easy way out for mother, but is it wise? We are only now beginning to see the effects on children who have been brought up in a television world. The present teen generation is the first to have been nurtured on TV since infancy, and it wants flashing-light shows, lulling drugs and incessant noise. Can't we at least dispense with TV at mealtime?

As for the games or play, they can wait. The child should come to the table with the rest of the family as a matter of discipline, whether he eats or not.

6) **Boredom with adult talk.** No one can expect mother and father to direct all their conversation to sensitive offspring. In fact, this would be ridiculous and unwise. But when all the talk is miles above the head of an only child, or even of two young children, naturally they feel left out. An effort should be made to bring them into the conversation now and then during the meal, with queries about play, or school, or even a favorite TV program.

Nor should a child be forced to sit at table until everyone else is completely finished. Good manners demand a request, "May I be excused?" but if this bit of politeness is observed, and if a reasonable effort has been made to finish the very small helpings on the child's plate and the milk in his glass, he should be permitted to depart to his own little world.

7) **The food offered is strange, he has never had it before.** No matter how delicious a new food may be, children by instinct shun from it. They will feel courageous enough to try it if other children around them are gobbling it up happily, or if they are so hungry they will accept it for lack of something better. They might be tempted to try it simply because an adored father eats it with gusto, but generally an adult's recommendation is not enough. Young children have not yet developed critical tastes. For the most part, they prefer bland, lightly seasoned food. Their liking for such sharp or spicily flavored foods as hot dogs and salami is because these foods can be eaten by hand—an attraction that makes up for taste.

But if the child's withdrawal from strange foods is pampered by providing a separate menu for him, he will never be encouraged to learn about new foods, and his eating habits will remain in a narrow rut.

When the father of the family is late getting home for dinner, or away from home frequently, feeding the children separately from grown-ups may be the only solution. But it's preferable, whenever possible, for them to be served the same foods as the rest of the family. The earlier they learn to adjust to a more varied diet, the better.

8) **The child has not had enough outdoor exercise.** One of the great drawbacks of TV is that it too often keeps children indoors when they should be playing outside in the open air. They grow accustomed to this soft, undemanding existence and, when they reach the teens,

they consider having to walk three blocks a terrible hardship.

TV is here to stay, we can't wish it out the window. But the wise parent will put a limit on the amount of time permitted for TV viewing and find ways to keep children occupied out of doors. With an only child, this may be far from easy. It may entail getting on the phone day after day to arrange playing time with other children. It may mean offering to take turns at baby-sitting with another mother. It may mean trips to skating rinks, or swimming pools, or public parks. Or it may mean becoming a Den Mother for budding Cub Scouts, or a leader for a Brownie troop. However much a bore such activities may be, just keep reminding yourself that being a parent has never been easy. You didn't think it would be, did you?

9) **He just finished snacking a half-hour before mealtime,**

OR

10) **He has been eating sweets and drinking cokes at a neighbor's most of the afternoon.** Ah, snacks! They are the bane of a parent's existence. Yet, like TV, they have become part of The American Way of Life. We have to live with them, so we might as well fit snack time into the day's menu pattern.

THE SNACKING SYNDROME: WHAT TO DO ABOUT IT

Accept this as an incontrovertible fact:

Snack foods that can be eaten by hand, impulsively, are much more interesting to youngsters than any others.

There's a wonderful freedom about opening the refrigerator door, looking at the selection on display, and taking what appeals to you. It's something like a visit to a Horn & Hardart Automat.

There are many nutritious ready-to-eat foods which can be kept in the refrigerator for snack meals. For instance:

- Fruit: apples, pears, blue plums, seedless white grapes, tangerines, bananas
- Yogurt in fruit flavors
- Homogenized or chocolate milk
- Juices: fruit juices and tomato juice
- Ice cream in Dixie cups (in the freezer)
- Cheese: mild soft cheese spreads or processed cheeses

Pantry shelf snacks might include:

- Raisins in individual packs
- Dried fruit (dates, apricots, prunes)
- Nuts (preferably in the shells)
- Graham crackers
- Fruit-filled cookies

The latter two are preferable to regular sugar cookies, the graham crackers because they are made with whole-wheat flour, the fruit-filled cookies because the dried fruit in them (usually raisins) is a good source of iron, calcium and Vitamin A.

Nuts are a protein food, used a great deal in vegetarian diets (some vegetarians exist on nothing more than nuts, fruit and raw vegetables) and are much to be preferred over potato or corn chips. The only drawback to having nuts on hand for snacks is that children fill up on them so quickly, because of the high fat content, that when regular mealtime arrives their appetite is dead. For this reason, nuts in the shell offer an advantage. They have not been salted and it takes time to remove the shells—which means fewer of the nuts will be eaten.

All the items suggested so far can be purchased ready to eat. In addition, when preparing for family use such foods as cup custards, milk puddings, fruited or plain gelatin or deviled eggs, it's wise to make up extras to keep around for snacks. Puddings and custards are especially nice for bedtime snacks.

Carrot sticks should also be ready at all times for impulse eating. These can be kept fresh in a sealed plastic bag for several days. Most children prefer carrot sticks to other raw vegetables, and carrots are loaded with important food elements—one of the best of all sources of Vitamin A, and a good source (when raw) of Vitamin C, calcium, phosphorus and potassium.

What about the other snack foods that are displayed so close to the supermarket check-out counter? The potato chips, cheese snacks, corn snacks, cookies, soft-drink mixes, candies and gum?

These all fall into the "empty calorie" classification. This means they have little nutritive value beyond their calorie count. They may serve as "quick energy," as the ads always remind us, but a child who is a finicky eater is better off getting that quick energy with foods which also provide something else of value. Raisins are as good a source of "quick energy" as candies; nuts have far more food value than potato chips; fruit juices certainly are more desirable than drinks made with mixes whose base is nothing more than sugar, artificial flavoring and coloring.

Then there is the question of soda pop. In the last decade, the U.S. Department of Agriculture tells us, Americans are drinking soft drinks more and milk less. Dentists are vehement in their opposition to sweet carbonated drinks, especially the cola drinks. Our dentist tells us he can tell how many cokes a young patient drinks by the number of cavities in his teeth. If the only soda drinkers in the family are the youngsters, one way of controlling their intake is to buy a minimum number of the 7-oz. bottles, say two per child per week, and when those have been consumed, no more will be permitted until the next week. If grown-ups like the same beverages, control becomes more difficult. It might be a good idea to lock up the soda supply, then dole out one bottle at a time under adult supervision.

For younger children, the toddlers and pre-schoolers, light snacks between meals are desirable and should definitely be planned for. The digestive systems of these smaller children can only handle limited quantities of food at a time and for this reason, five very light meals a day are far better than three larger ones. The snack meal may be nothing more than fruit juice and a fruit-filled cookie, or a cup of flavored yogurt, but the younger child should have something—and it should not be candy or soda.

After-school snacking is to be expected from children of all ages. To have a snack is part of the lure of coming home. This is when a few hard-cooked or deviled eggs are consumed with delight, or a chocolate pudding, or cheese and crackers.

The one time when snacking should be firmly discouraged is just before dinner. And this is when it's most likely to occur—especially when dinner must be delayed until seven o'clock or later, waiting for daddy to get home.

Before-dinner snacks should be vegetable relishes (carrot sticks, celery, olives) or fruit or tomato juice. These are appetizers; they help to allay hunger without taking the edge off appetite. Far better to encourage nibbling on foods such as these than to find your darling wolfing down chocolate bars a half-hour before you plan to put dinner on the table.

FINICKY TEEN-AGERS

A normal, healthy teen-age boy eats three times as much as his father. If your male teen-ager doesn't wolf down fantastic quantities of food, it could be because of emotional disturbance (puppy love, worry over school work, or possibly because he feels left out of the "in" crowd). Or maybe he gorges on sodas, hamburgers, French fries and candy bars at the local sweet shop every afternoon. Or he could be smoking too much. Or—and this is a factor no longer to be overlooked—he may be hung up on "pot."

Teen-age girls, by contrast, even the perfectly healthy specimens, often eat less than they did when ten or eleven. But if they are such fussy eaters that most of the food is regularly left on their plates, or if they skip meals altogether, there *is* cause for alarm, for they need proper nutrition now if they are to be the mothers of healthy children later.

The dieting fad is often the reason for a teen-age girl skipping meals. She believes that by doing without breakfast and possibly lunch as well, she will look like one of those skinny models who lead such seemingly glamorous lives. Actually, controlled tests have proved that teen-age girls who skip breakfast entirely are more likely to be overweight than those who eat a nutritious breakfast. In one such test in Iowa, this was found to be true of girls whose total calorie intake for the day was *less* than that of another group on a controlled, well-balanced diet. Perhaps it's a question of the body burning up certain foods faster than others (this is the theory behind the high protein diet), or that more roughage in the diet contributes to better elimination. In any case, the best reducing diet is one that is nutritionally well-balanced—and if your teen-age daughter is concerned about spreading hips or a spare tire around her midriff, she should know this. She should also be reminded frequently that outdoor exercise is just as important in a reducing regime as limited food intake.

Appealing to vanity is usually the most effective way to reach teen-agers, because this is the age when both boys and girls are painfully conscious of their looks. Complexion troubles can be traced directly to poor eating habits, just as can overweight. Outdoor exercise will help to provoke better appetite, get rid of flabby fat, and may also help to relieve those emotional problems.

And the emotional problems are not to be ignored. Teen-agers are traditionally reluctant to discuss personal affairs with parents, but the school guidance counselor may be able to draw them out, or consult your family doctor—or a psychiatrist. (Many localities now maintain special clinics for teen-agers where both group therapy and individual consultation are available at moderate cost.)

An outsider may be much more convincing than you can be in persuading your teen-ager to follow a proper diet, too. With teen-agers, the longest way 'round is often the shortest way to the point. If the home economics teacher at school, or your doctor, or the baseball coach can get the nutrition story across, you may find your teen-ager suddenly is finicky in demanding more of the good-for-you foods—and if *that* happens, do be indulgent.

SHORT GUIDE TO NUTRITION

Every day's menu should include some of the following in the amounts indicated:

The Basic Four

1. **Meat or meat substitutes**

   2 or more of the following:

   beef, lamb, veal, pork, ham, liver, tongue, poultry, fish, cheese, nuts, or legumes (beans and peas)

2. **Milk products or their equivalents**

   3 cups daily for children
   4 cups daily for teen-agers

Not all of this need be consumed as a beverage. When milk (or instant nonfat dry milk) is used in cooking, or cottage cheese added to salads or served up in a soufflé or pie, or ice cream or milk sherbets served for snacks or desserts, these can be counted part of the daily milk allotment.

(If a child's system is upset by whole milk, a special formula drink can be obtained through your pediatrician. Some children bothered by whole milk can take nonfat dry milk in cooked or processed foods. Some bothered by cow's milk can drink goat's milk—if they will!)

3. **Vegetables and fruits**

   4 or more servings of the following:

   at least one citrus fruit, tomato or raw vegetable; and yellow or green vegetables such as carrots, spinach, broccoli, green beans, sweet potatoes

4. **Bread, cereals, other grains**

 4 or more servings of:

 whole grain cereal products (whole wheat, rye, cornmeal, bran, oatmeal) or enriched flours or bread

"Enriched" grain products (breads, breakfast cereals, flours) are those that first have been refined—which removes the health-giving bran and with it important minerals and vitamins—then have had some (but not all) of the deleted vitamins and minerals put back in again. "Enriched" products are preferable to those that have been merely refined, but the products which have not been so highly refined in the first place are still better. The grains are important as the chief source of Vitamin B and B Complex (see following chart).

Vitamin-Mineral Chart

Vitamin	Source	Importance in Diet
A	carrots spinach turnip greens sweet potatoes beet greens squash cantaloupe liver liverwurst butter and margarine egg yolk	good for eyes (especially in adjustment to light changes), for skin and complexion, and helps to resist nasal infections

Vitamin	Source	Importance in Diet
B_1,* B_2,† B_{12},‡ B Complex	liver whole-grain cereals enriched or fortified breads and flours meats, *esp.* pork fish milk peanuts egg yolk yeast tablets	needed for steady nerves and alert mind, to help appetite and digestion, to resist infection, and to convert carbohydrates and fats to body use
C §	citrus fruits tomatoes oranges strawberries sweet potatoes liver most raw vegetables and fruits	necessary for sound teeth and gums; helps prevent easy bleeding
D	sunlight (out of doors) egg yolk fortified milk fish liver oil oily fish, tuna, mackerel	helps in absorption of and utilization of calcium, for strong bones and teeth
E	butter and margarine vegetable oils beans and peas wheat germ egg yolk nuts leafy vegetables	needed for reproduction and growth
K	green leafy and root vegetables fruits vegetable oils	needed for normal blood clotting

* Also called thiamin. † Also called riboflavin. ‡ Also called niacin. § Also called ascorbic acid.

Mineral	Source	Importance in Diet
calcium	milk cheese egg yolk green leafy vegetables carrots salmon sardines broccoli whole grain or enriched bread and cereals dried legumes nuts	needed for building bones and teeth; helps regulate nerve and muscle action and in blood clotting
phosphorus	milk cheese egg yolk lean meats legumes (beans and peas) carrots potatoes	needed for building bones and teeth and to utilize proteins, fats, and carbohydrates in the body
iron	liver turkey meats eggs legumes nuts green leafy vegetables prunes green peas	helps provide energy; carries oxygen from lungs to rest of body
sodium	salt corned beef fish cheese bread and cereals	helps maintain water balance in body; needed for muscle contraction

Common Sense About Vitamins and Minerals

Giving a child vitamin pills is *not* going to increase his appetite. In fact, under normal circumstances, if the child's diet is well-balanced there is no need for vitamin pills. It is far better for the child to get these essential food elements in the natural way, in food, than in the form of pills. Only when a child is malnourished or sickly are vitamin pills recommended as a therapeutic measure, and then they should be given only because your doctor recommends it.

Milk enriched with Vitamin D is recommended, but most commercially bottled milk today is so enriched. Besides, the best of all sources of Vitamin D is sunlight, absorbed out of doors, in the open air.

If a child is allergic to milk, calcium tablets might be a good thing, though still better is to give the child as many other foods which are a good source of calcium as possible. Check the Vitamin-Mineral Chart to see which foods so qualify.

An anemic child may need liver pills or iron pills—but again, give these only upon recommendation by your doctor, and try in any case to include iron-rich foods frequently in the diet.

For the vast majority of children (and adults, too), nutritious food is the best source of vitamins, minerals and all other essential food elements.

Proteins, Carbohydrates and Fats

There is virtually no food which is pure protein, or pure carbohydrate, or pure fat. Most foods contain some of all three, in varying proportions. And all of us need all three of these food components every day—in varying proportions.

The foods that are highest in protein content are the meats, fish, poultry, cheese and milk. Nuts and whole-grain products also are excellent sources of protein—but a different type of protein, one that is called "incomplete" because the body cannot absorb it unless combined in the diet with some of the "complete" proteins.

Protein is essential for growth and repair, what is sometimes called "body maintenance." Also, it gives *lasting* energy as compared to the *quick* energy of high-carbohydrate foods. A child who has had an egg for breakfast will have more bounce and pep all morning (and be more attentive in school) than one whose breakfast consisted only of toast and juice.

The foods that are highest in *carbohydrates* are the sugars and starches. These are the cheapest as well as the most easily and quickly digested form of fuel for the human body. But when sugars and starches are eaten in excessive amounts, they tend to satisfy energy needs so quickly that little or no appetite is left for other foods which are more important nutritionally.

Certain of these high carbohydrate foods have little else to offer *but* quick energy—sugar candies, gum and carbonated drinks, for example. Others, such as enriched or whole grain breads, do give the body essential food needs. Fruits and vegetables, which are also high-carbohydrate foods, provide elements which the body must have *every day*.

The foods highest in *fat* are butter, margarine, fat meats, cream, oil, cheeses and oily fish. Our bodies must have a certain degree of fat every day, but Americans consume a higher proportion of fats and oils than any other people in the world, so a conscientious American mother rarely needs to worry about whether there is enough fat in her child's diet. The opposite is more likely to be true, especially as so many of the snack foods (potato chips, salted nuts, cheese spreads and sour cream dips) are high-fat content foods. Excess fat in the diet tends to deaden appetite for other more needed foods—and besides, it's bad for the complexion. Animal fats (butter, lard, bacon drippings and fat meat) are also hard to digest, more likely to cause stomach upsets (which in turn may lead to untouched food) and may contribute to constipation.

FOOD ALLERGIES, COMMON AND UNCOMMON

Young children seem to be even more subject to allergies than adults, and the most common *food allergies* include those foods absolutely essential to a well-balanced diet: milk, eggs, oranges, wheat. If your child is allergic to any one of these, you have a difficult role ahead, because you must seek other ways to provide the essential food elements contained in the foods to which he is sensitive.

Poor appetite in itself is no indication of an allergy, but a child who has an allergy may be lacking in appetite, simply because his allergy prevents him from feeling well. The most obvious symptoms of an allergy are eczema (skin rashes), hives, asthma, runny nose, headaches, and gastro-intestinal disturbances.

The allergy is due to some quirk in the child's physical make-up, but the effects will be more severe if the child is disturbed emotionally or is tense, nervous or worried. Conversely, the allergy will bother him less if he is relaxed, happy, has had plenty of sleep and outdoor exercise (provided, of course, that being outdoors does not expose him to elements in the atmosphere to which he is allergic).

Any allergy, even allergies to ragweed, dust, smoke or exhaust fumes, can interfere with appetite and general health, but food allergies are more of a problem because the child must follow a special diet—which is bound to make the child still more finicky and difficult about food, if that is possible.

How do you know whether your child has an allergy? The scratch test is less effective in determining food allergies than the diet elimination test. The tests are carried out under the supervision of a physician, but it is possible for a mother to try the diet test on her own. I did, in desperation, after visits to one specialist after another failed to determine the cause of my daughter's almost daily severe stomach cramps (often so bad she was unable to go to school). I suspected milk might be the cause, because she had had colic as a baby, so we first tried eliminating whole milk, then all milk, including nonfat dry milk—and the stomach cramps went away. After total elimination of milk in all forms for a period of several months, she was able, gradually, once again to take milk and milk products in moderate degrees. However, she will never be able to consume milk products as freely as most other people do and periodically she must go on a milkless diet for a brief period.

The most common food allergies are these (more or less in this order of incidence):

wheat
eggs
milk and milk products
oranges
fish
chocolate
honey
tomatoes
strawberries
garlic
onion
corn and all corn products (including corn oil)
cabbage

To carry out the elimination test, *completely* eliminate one food at a time from the diet for one week. If the symptoms go away, you have a clue, at least. If they do not go away, try eliminating the next food on the list. And so on. Not infrequently a child will be allergic to more than one food.

You may already have observed that certain foods tend to cause stomach upsets. Any food which frequently causes an upset should be eliminated, even though this may not be strictly an allergic reaction. It may be only a food which your child finds difficult to digest—and remember that the digestive system of younger children is much more delicate than that of adults.

What do you do if you find your child is allergic to wheat, for example? Can he ever eat a wheat product again in his life? Yes, eventually. Some people outgrow childhood allergies completely when they become adults.

If the child has an allergy, the sooner you are aware of it the better, for the longer the poisonous effects build up in his body, the harder it will be for him to throw off the effects.

Once you know what the allergy is, eliminate the food completely from the diet for a period of at least a month, preferably longer. Then, very gradually, let him have a very small amount—perhaps once a week at first, then every few days. When the allergic symptoms return, you will know that he has passed the level of tolerance and once again you have to eliminate the food completely.

Wheat and milk are the most difficult of the allergies to adjust to. Mothers faced with a wheat allergy must search out health stores carrying rice flour, rye flour, potato flour and so on. Such stores usually carry breads made with these grains, too. You will find to your distress that commercial cornbreads or cornbread mixes will not do, because they are made partially with wheat flour. The same is true of commercial rye and pumpernickel bread. You will have to start reading labels on *all* commercial products to make sure the offending food ingredient is not included.

Parents dealing with milk allergies today have it easier than I did ten years ago. Baker's bread must be eliminated (except the Italian and French breads), but it may be possible to buy kosher bread. It would be well to seek out a kosher grocery, since Orthodox Jewish dietary laws forbid milk and meat products to be consumed in the same meal—therefore a large selection of foods which contain no milk are available in such shops.

Some corn oil margarines contain no dry milk at all, but beware of frankfurters (hot dogs cannot be purchased at roadside stands), commercial cookies, and many frozen ready-to-heat products which have been "enriched" with nonfat dry milk.

Ice cream is out (you will grow to dread the tinkling bell of the Good Humor man, since your little one can't join the other neighborhood children at his wagon), so are puddings, éclairs, many other desserts, to say nothing of macaroni and cheese, cream puddings, and all kinds of cheeses and cheese spread.

It isn't fun. The child may have to give up some of his favorite foods, and that will make mealtime still more of an ordeal. But it can be done.

And never forget the psychological factor. A relaxed, happy, busy child, free from tensions or worries, is not nearly as bothered by his allergies, no matter how many he may have, as the worried, unhappy, or insecure child.

BELLYACHES, AND WHAT TO DO ABOUT THEM

A stomach ache may be caused by any one of many factors, physiological or psychological, but because this could be the first symptom of a serious illness it should not be ignored.

Sometimes the cause is obvious. For example, when the child has bolted down his food, a bellyache often follows immediately. Gulping down food without properly chewing it sends it into the digestive stream like rocks into a drain pipe. This may have happened because the child wants to go out to play, or is "starved"—and even finicky eaters frequently have such spells. The finicky eater may also suffer because he is angered if you should insist he eat something he doesn't want to eat. This kind of stomach ache can be intensely painful, but it usually passes away within a short time.

Stomach aches caused by simple gas pains, often called "heartburn," are also the result of improper digestion. Certain foods are more likely to lead to stomach gas than others: cabbage, onions, dried beans, very cold milk, or too much milk at once.

A child who has a tendency toward frequent gas pains (and some individuals by nature are more bothered by this tendency than others) should avoid such foods, or have them in limited quantities. Milk is less likely to cause gas pains when cooked in puddings, sauces, or casseroles.

Ice-cold drinks also can cause gas pains, especially if drunk in quantity on a very hot day. Candy gobbled down between meals sometimes causes stomach cramps, too. And fried foods, especially if breaded before frying, are notoriously conducive to gas formation.

But stomach aches can also be brought on by emotional stress. Nagging about what a child has or has not eaten could cause a bellyache. Arguments between parents at the table is a frequent cause. Being forced to play with children whom he dislikes (or he fears do not like him) might also bring on a stomach cramp. Just having to go to school could bring on such pain if the situation to be faced at school is a worrisome one for any of a dozen reasons.

When your child has a stomach ache, the first thing to do is to determine the cause. If it's simply due to overeating, or improper eating, the best thing is to have him lie down for at least a half-hour. By that time the cramps should have subsided.

If pains are caused by any particular foods to which he has a sensitivity, naturally you will try to eliminate such foods from his diet in future. Cucumbers, green peppers, radishes, garlic and turnips are all vegetables that cause indigestion in some people.

If the cause of the stomach aches is emotional, you will have to play it cool, trying to discover the underlying unhappiness and helping him to get better perspective on his relations to others.

But any time a stomach ache persists, or recurs regularly, be sure to consult the doctor, remembering it could be a danger signal.

WAYS TO SNEAK NUTRITION INTO FAVORITE FOODS

When your finicky one's poor appetite makes it seem all but impossible to work the minimum Basic Four requirements into the day's menu, try sneaking some extra nutrition into those foods he likes best.

For example, "enrich" his hamburgers, puddings and milk drinks with added nonfat dry milk. In the case of hamburgers, the dry milk is worked into the meat along with salt. The hamburgers taste just the same—but the milk is there, to be eaten instead of drunk.

Milk drinks (eggnog, chocolate milk, strawberry frosted, etc.) become "double milk drinks" by adding whole milk to nonfat dry milk. The nonfat dry milk is dissolved in the whole milk also before the latter is added to cream sauce or to puddings. Nonfat dry milk can even be added to spaghetti sauce without changing the taste or appearance.

Spaghetti sauce can also be enriched with grated American cheese added shortly before the sauce is removed from the heat.

Hot cooked breakfast cereals, oatmeal, cream of wheat and so on, can be made with milk instead of water as the liquid—and they are creamier and taste far better this way, too.

Add more fruit to the diet by topping breakfast cereal with fresh, canned or dried fruit: peaches, strawberries, sliced bananas, raisins, canned sliced apples, applesauce, blueberries or raspberries (in season). Use chopped sugared fresh fruit as ice cream toppings—or chopped drained canned fruit (such as peaches and plums) over puddings.

Vegetables can be sneaked into sauces without the child even knowing it. When making spaghetti sauce, for example, sauté grated carrots and onion in the oil first, then add tomatoes (or prepared tomato sauce). A recipe for this Vege-Tomato Sauce for Spaghetti will be found on page 104.

The same trick can be followed in making gravy for pot roast or stews. Minced or grated vegetables, carrots, celery, onions and tomatoes, are simmered in the pan drippings until very soft, then liquid is added. This is what is called in French a *mirepoix.* The vegetables actually thicken the sauce so that no flour is needed, and the flavor is far, far better than that of ordinary gravy.

Cole slaw is usually more appealing than cooked cabbage—and cole slaw to which grated carrot has been added may turn out to be even more popular than the usual kind. (See page 111.)

The eternally popular Golden Glow Salad, a mixture of grated carrot and crushed pineapple in gelatin, is another sly way of getting your finicky one to eat carrots without even knowing it.

Eggs beaten into nogs (recipes for a number of these will be found in the section on drinks) may be much more attractive than fried eggs for breakfast. Most children are fond of deviled eggs, and sliced eggs on potato chips make an excellent snack or before-dinner appetizer. (Grown-ups will like these, too.)

If whole wheat or cracked wheat bread does not appeal to your finicky one, steamed Boston brown bread may, and it is made with molasses (an excellent source of iron), whole wheat and rye flours, and cornmeal—a terrific lot of nutrition in one loaf. This can be purchased in cans. It also makes fine sandwiches when spread with a cream cheese and chopped-nut filling.

Recipes for Bran Muffins, Graham Gems, Honey Buns (made with brown sugar, nuts and raisins) and a Brown Fruit Bread (made with whole wheat, brown sugar, chopped fruit, nuts and orange juice) will be found in the recipe section. (Check the Index to locate recipes.) All these contain whole grain cereals. In addition, there are many commercial mixes for bran muffins, corn muffins and so on, to be found in every supermarket.

Some children like salads very much, others won't touch them. If your problem eater is a salad-resister, try slipping tomato slices into hamburgers, put lettuce in sandwiches, and always keep carrot and celery sticks on hand.

Keep in mind, too, that hand-to-mouth foods have a special appeal to children. A salad in the hand (encased in a bun) may be worth two on the plate. Look at the Hero's phenomenal success: it's salad, meat, cheese, what-have-you, a meal between chunks of bread.

PART II

MENUS

Where dishes or drinks appear in bold type, recipes will be found elsewhere in the book. Consult the Index.

Breakfast

Children do not demand, expect or want variety at the breakfast table. If certain foods are favorites with them at breakfast time, you may give them the same breakfast day after day—if that is their preference. It's also the one meal when you can indulge their fancies, as long as they receive adequate nutrition.

I can recall a time when my daughter wanted hot soup for breakfast—tomato soup one morning, chicken-noodle soup another. The fancy was short-lived, but since both these soups are nourishing, I gave in to her whims. These soups have been included in two of the following menus. They are especially good for late breakfasts on weekends, when breakfast is really brunch.

Eggnog

Favorite cold cereal topped with berries

* * *

Juice

Fried Egg on Toast

Cocoa topped with marshmallow

* * *

Hot cream of tomato soup
Bacon sandwich
(crisp bacon between slices of whole wheat toast)

* * *

Banana Orange Nog

Cinnamon toast

* * *

Orange juice

Animal Pancakes

* * *

Pineapple-orange juice
Scrambled Eggs

Honey Buns

* * *

Grapefruit

French Toast

Milk or Cocoa

* * *

Cream of chicken soup

Toasted corn muffins or sticks with jam

* * *

Juice

Enriched Scrambled Egg

Raisin toast

* * *

Orange juice

Enriched Oatmeal with Raisins

* * *

Melon slice

Pineapple Corn Muffins

Lunch

The first six of the following menus can be sent to school in a lunch box. The last ones are more suitable for lunches served at home.

Lunch-box Combinations

Ham and Swiss cheese on rye
Sweet gherkin pickles
Raisin cookies
Milk (in thermos, or purchased at school)

* * *

Salami-Cream Cheese Sandwich

Carrot sticks in a plastic bag
Orange cup cake
Milk

* * *

Peanut butter and jelly sandwich
Apple

Deviled Eggs

* * *

Bologna-Cottage Cheese Sandwich

Blue plums or banana
Chocolate milk
Box of raisins

* * *

Egg Salad Sandwich

Milk
Gingerbread

* * *

Cream cheese-nut sandwich on Boston brown bread
Tangerine or banana
Milk

* * *

At-home Lunches

Grilled Cheese Sandwich

Fruit juice
Rice pudding with raisins

* * *

Chicken noodle soup
Hot dog
Instant chocolate pudding
Milk

* * *

Tuna salad
Toasted English muffins
Pineapple tapioca pudding

* * *

Cream of mushroom soup
Cheese and tomato sandwich on cracked wheat
Ice cream

* * *

Cheese Eggs on Toast

Fresh pear or other fruit
Milk or Cocoa

Afternoon Snacks

All the snacks for which recipes are provided can be prepared by the children themselves—a good way to encourage interest in eating.

Fruit Salad in Gelatin
Cookies
Chocolate milk

* * *

Deviled Eggs
Orange Nog

* * *

Egg Slices on Potato Chips
Carrot sticks, stuffed olives
Ginger ale or cola drink

* * *

Applesauce
Frosted Chocolate
Graham crackers

* * *

Peach pudding
Orange juice and ginger ale

* * *

Fruit-flavored yogurt
Peanut Butter Squares

* * *

Peach-Lime-Lemon Float
Easy Coconut Macaroons

* * *

Cheese Dreams
Pineapple Nog

* * *

Applewiches

Strawberry Cow

* * *

Bananas Rolled in Coconut

Purple Cow Nog

* * *

Favorite cheese spread and crackers

Pineapple Ice Cream Soda

* * *

Graham Cracker Milk Shake

Fresh fruit

Dinner

As a matter of principle, children should be expected to eat the same food as their parents at dinner—especially when they sit at the same table. However, for those families which must have two separate dinner hours (when father arrives home too late for the children's mealtime) and for the evenings when father is away, or when both parents plan to go out for dinner, it's best to prepare food which suits children's special wants and needs.

The following menus are all planned especially for children with typical children's tastes in mind. Make portions very small for the finicky eaters. For the dishes which cannot be prepared for one child, or even for two children with poor appetites, use the remaining portions to make future TV dinners, placing individual portions on sectioned aluminum foil plates (these can be purchased in housewares departments), wrap plates in plastic bags to freeze. Such homemade TV dinners are usually much tastier than the commercial combinations.

* * *

Cheeseburger
Pickles and relishes
Sliced tomatoes with Russian dressing
Ice cream, chocolate sauce
Milk

* * *

Pork chops
(cut meat from bone for younger children)
Candied sweet potatoes
Green beans
Canned peaches with cream
Milk

* * *

Creole Meat Balls and Rice

Carrot sticks
Raspberry Sundae
(frozen raspberries over ice cream)
Milk

* * *

Broiled chicken
Noodles
Spinach or broccoli
Baked cup custard

* * *

Sliced roast meat heated in gravy
Mashed potato
Stewed tomatoes
Raspberry gelatin with whipped topping
Milk

* * *

Cream of tomato soup
Baked beans and frankfurters
Celery and olives
Blueberry pie
Milk

* * *

Baked Cheese Fondue

Green peas   Corn muffins
Strawberries with cream

* * *

Tomato-topped Macaroni and Cheese

Kernel corn
Cucumbers with French or Italian dressing
Butterscotch pudding (from mix)
Milk

* * *

Chicken or Tuna à la King

Broccoli or asparagus
French fries (frozen)
Apple crisp (from mix)
Milk

* * *

Scrambled Eggs and Frankfurters

Mixed vegetables (frozen)
Small baked potato
Tomato and lettuce salad
Milk   Cookies or cake

* * *

Minute steak
Cottage-fried Potatoes

Green or lima beans
Carrot sticks

Gingerbread with whipped cream topping
Milk

* * *

Spaghetti with Vege-Tomato Sauce

Hearts of lettuce with child's favorite dressing
Instant vanilla pudding

Milk

* * *

Won-ton soup (frozen)

Baked Cheese Fondue

French fries (frozen)

Braised Celery

Ice cream
Milk

* * *

Baked Tuna Chow Mein

Escalloped Tomatoes

Cole slaw
Milk Cookies

RECIPES

Drinks

Young people love to experiment, so put out the fixings, let them mix up their own drinks—with suggestions from you. For older children and teen-agers, an electric blender is a great help in beating up the frosteds and frappés, though younger children should not be permitted to use the blender because of the danger of fingers getting in the way of blades still in motion. For the under-10s, an ordinary rotary beater is safer and just as much fun. For the sodas made with bottled carbonated drinks and ice cream out of the freezer, nothing more is needed than a long-handled ice tea spoon for beating the ice cream into the carbonated beverage.

Juice Combinations and Floats

PINEAPPLE-LEMON FLOAT

Fill tall tumblers a little more than half full with canned pineapple juice. To each glass add a scoop of lemon sherbet. Fill glass with club soda or ginger ale. Add a cherry for garnish.

STRAWBERRY FLOAT

Make pink lemonade with frozen concentrate. Pour the pink lemonade into glasses or paper cups. Put a scoop of strawberry ice cream in each. Beat with long-handled spoon just to partially melt ice cream. Drink through straws.

ORANGE PINEAPPLE PUNCH

First, make frozen pineapple cubes by pouring canned pineapple juice into an ice tray. This needs to be done a day ahead. Remove the pineapple cubes from the ice tray exactly as plain ice is removed, add the pineapple cubes to glasses of orange juice. Garnish each drink with a maraschino cherry.

RASPBERRY LEMON PUNCH

Save the syrup from frozen raspberries. Make lemonade with a 6-ounce can of frozen lemonade concentrate; to this add ½ cup raspberry syrup (or as much as there is available). Stir to blend well, then pour in contents of a 7-ounce bottle of club soda or lime-lemon carbonated drink. This makes enough for 6 to 8 drinks (depending on size of paper cups or glasses).

TANGERINE FLOAT

Add water to frozen tangerine juice concentrate as directed (or use canned tangerine juice). Pour into tall glasses or paper cups. Add a scoop of vanilla ice cream to each and beat with long-handled spoon enough to partially melt ice cream. Drink through straws.

PEACH-LIME-LEMON FLOAT

Add water to lime-lemonade frozen concentrate as directed. Pour into glasses or paper cups. Add a scoop of peach ice cream to each, beat with long-handled spoon just enough to partially melt ice cream. Drink through straws.

GINGER GRAPE

Combine equal parts grape juice (canned, or frozen reconstituted) and ginger ale. Serve this way with ice cubes, or add a scoop of vanilla ice cream to each.

ORANGE SPRITZER

Fill glasses half full with orange juice. Add ice cubes and spirals of orange peel. Fill glasses with club soda. Very refreshing—grown-ups will like it, too.

Homemade Sodas

BROWN COW

Place a scoop of vanilla or chocolate ice cream in a tall glass. Pour in root beer and stir briskly with a long-handled spoon until the ice cream is about half melted. (Or do this in an electric blender, but beat no more than 30 seconds—too much beating will make it a frappé rather than an ice cream soda.) Drink through straws.

STRAWBERRY COW

Place 1 pint of strawberry ice cream in a large mixing bowl, or the bowl of an electric mixer or electric blender. Add 2 cups of milk. Beat until foamy. Pour into tall glasses, filling half full. Add ginger ale, stir briskly. Drink through straws.

CREAM AND COLA

Place a scoop of vanilla ice cream in tall glass. Add bottled cola drink, stir briskly until ice cream is partially melted. Drink through straws.

RASPBERRY SODA

Place a scoop of raspberry milk sherbet, or black raspberry ice cream, in tall glass. Fill glass with ginger ale. Stir briskly until ice cream is nearly all melted. Drink through straw.

PINEAPPLE ICE CREAM SODA

For each serving, place scoop of pineapple ice cream in a glass, add ½ cup milk, stir briskly, then add ginger ale or club soda and stir until foamy. (Or, use vanilla ice cream and pineapple juice instead of milk.)

The Nog Family

PLAIN EGGNOG

(1 Serving)

1 egg
1 cup milk
½ teaspoon vanilla extract
1 tablespoon sugar (or to taste)
Dash of nutmeg

Combine all ingredients in a bowl and beat with rotary beater until foamy; or beat in electric blender 60 seconds. This makes an excellent "instant breakfast" for finicky school children.

FORTIFIED EGGNOG

(1 Serving)

1 egg
⅓ cup instant dry milk
1 tablespoon sugar (or to taste)
⅔ cup whole milk
½ teaspoon vanilla extract
Dash of nutmeg or cinnamon

Place egg, instant milk, sugar and half the whole milk in bowl or blender. Beat just to blend. Add remaining milk and vanilla. Beat until foamy. Top with nutmeg or cinnamon. A good way to increase milk intake for a child who doesn't care much for milk.

DIETER'S EGGNOG

For weight-conscious teen-age girls

(1 Serving)

1 egg
⅓ cup instant dry milk
⅔ cup skimmed milk or water
½ teaspoon vanilla
Noncaloric sweetener to taste

Combine ingredients in bowl or blender, beat until foamy. An excellent "instant breakfast."

CHOCOLATE EGGNOG

(1 Serving)

1 egg
1 cup chocolate milk
½ to 1 teaspoon vanilla (to taste)
¼ teaspoon cinnamon

Combine all ingredients, beat until foamy. This may appeal to children who don't care much for plain eggnog. If this amount of cinnamon is too strong, use less, or add a dash of nutmeg instead.

SPICY CHRISTMAS EGGNOG

(10 Servings)

8 eggs, separated
⅓ cup sugar
½ teaspoon cinnamon
¼ teaspoon cloves
¼ teaspoon nutmeg
2 teaspoons vanilla
2 quarts milk

Beat together the egg yolks, sugar, spices and vanilla. Add the milk a cup at a time, beating until foamy. Separately beat the egg whites until stiff. Fold egg whites into the milk-egg mixture. Serve in paper cups from a punch bowl. (*With cut-out Christmas cookies, this makes a festive drink for a holiday children's or teen's party.*)

PINEAPPLE NOG

(1 Serving)

1 cup pineapple juice
1 egg
¼ cup light cream (or small scoop vanilla ice cream)

Combine egg and pineapple juice, beat until foamy; add cream or ice cream and beat just to blend well.

PURPLE COW NOG

(1 Serving)

¾ cup (6-oz. can) frozen grape juice concentrate
1 egg
1 tablespoon sugar
¾ cup milk
¼ teaspoon vanilla

Combine all ingredients (do not add water to grape juice concentrate); beat until foamy.

ORANGE NOG I

(1 Serving)

1 cup orange juice
1 teaspoon sugar
1 egg
¼ teaspoon vanilla
¼ cup milk or light cream
Dash of nutmeg

Combine all ingredients; beat until foamy.

ORANGE NOG II

(4 Servings)

1 6-oz. can orange juice concentrate
½ cup instant nonfat dry milk
3 eggs
2 cups water
½ teaspoon vanilla
Dash of nutmeg

Combine all ingredients but nutmeg, beat only until juice concentrate and dry milk are dissolved. Serve at once, sprinkled with nutmeg.

BANANA-ORANGE NOG

(1 Serving)

½ banana, peeled
1 tablespoon sugar
1 cup orange juice
1 egg
Pinch of cinnamon

If a rotary beater is used, cut banana in small pieces, beat until soft; add remaining ingredients, beat until smooth and foamy. If a blender is used, cut banana in cubes, place in blender with all remaining ingredients at once, beat until foamy.

Milk Shakes

GRAHAM CRACKER MILK SHAKE

(1 Serving)

4 graham crackers
1 cup milk
1 scoop vanilla ice cream

Soak crackers in milk until soft; add ice cream, beat until smooth. (*For extra nutrition, add an egg, making it a Graham Cracker Nog.*)

FROSTED CHOCOLATE

(2 Servings)

2 scoops chocolate ice cream
1 scoop vanilla ice cream
2 cups chocolate milk
Dash of cinnamon or nutmeg
Whipped topping mix

If rotary beater is to be used, let ice cream soften slightly at room temperature, then combine with milk and cinnamon and beat until smooth. If a blender is used, put ice cream right from freezer into blender with milk and cinnamon, beat until smooth. Serve topped with whipped topping (from pressurized can). Drink through straw, finish with spoon.

VANILLA MINT FRAPPÉ
(2 Servings)

2 scoops vanilla ice cream
¼ cup tiny candy mints
2 cups milk
Few drops green food coloring

This can only be made successfully in a blender. Put milk and candy into blender first, beat until candy is crushed and dissolved, then add ice cream and beat until smooth and foamy. Pour into tall glasses to serve; drink through straws.

Hot Drinks

HOT SPICED CIDER
(About 10 Servings)

4 cups sweet cider
½ teaspoon cinnamon
¼ teaspoon nutmeg
Pinch of powdered cloves
⅓ cup brown sugar

Combine ingredients, heat to steaming (do not boil). Serve in mugs.

JUNIOR GLOGG
(10 Servings)

When grown-ups are enjoying alcoholic drinks during the holiday season, this makes an appetizing hot punch for the younger generation.

1 can (6 oz.) frozen raspberry-lemon punch, reconstituted; or 4 cups Hawaiian Punch
1 can (6 oz.) frozen lemonade, reconstituted
¼ cup raisins
¼ teaspoon cinnamon
Pinch of cloves
1 orange, sliced
12 whole cloves

Combine raspberry-lemon punch (or Hawaiian Punch) with lemonade, raisins, cinnamon and cloves. Heat to steaming. Serve from a 2-quart bowl. Float orange slices stuck with whole cloves in punch for garnish.

Hand-To-Mouth Snacks

DEVILED EGGS

(3 to 6 Servings)

3 eggs, hard-cooked
2 tablespoons mayonnaise
¼ teaspoon prepared mustard
Dash of salt (from shaker)
Dash of pepper (from shaker)
Dash of paprika

To hard-cook eggs, place in a saucepan with hot water, enough water to cover eggs. Cover pan, cook over *moderate* heat until water comes to a boil, then turn heat as low as possible. Simmer 5 minutes, turn off heat, let eggs cool in the water. Pour off water, add cold water, let eggs stand in this for 5 minutes. When eggs are completely cold, remove the shells. (This method ensures the shells coming off easily, leaving eggs intact.) Cut eggs into halves carefully; remove yolks.

Break up yolks with a fork, add mayonnaise, mustard, salt and pepper, but keep mixture light and fluffy. Pile egg yolk mixture into the whites. Sprinkle paprika over top. Chill.

To pack deviled eggs in lunch box: wrap each half first in plastic wrap, then in foil. If foil is crinkled, so much the better —this will help prevent eggs from being mashed by other foods in the lunch box.

HAM-STUFFED EGGS

Prepare as for Deviled Eggs but add 2 tablespoons minced cooked ham to the yolk mixture. Instead of paprika, sprinkle minced parsley over the top of each egg half.

NUT-STUFFED EGGS

Prepare as for Deviled Eggs, but omit mustard, add 2 tablespoons finely-chopped peanuts, walnuts or almonds to the yolk mixture. Save one nut half for the top of each.

PEANUT BUTTER EGGS

Omit mustard from Deviled Eggs, add 2 tablespoons smooth or chunky peanut butter to egg yolks with mayonnaise.

CHEESE-STUFFED EGGS

3 eggs, hard-cooked
1 tablespoon soft Cheddar-type cheese spread
1 tablespoon soft or whipped margarine
¼ teaspoon prepared mustard
Paprika

Hard-cook eggs (see Deviled Eggs). To yolks, add cheese spread and margarine. Fill egg whites with this mixture. Sprinkle paprika over top.

EGG SLICES ON POTATO CHIPS

Hard-cook eggs as previously described. When cold, remove the shells. Slice with an egg-slicer. Serve egg slices on large firm potato chips as an appetizer.

COTTAGE CHEESE STUFFED CELERY

Trim celery sticks and cut into 2-inch lengths. Pile cottage cheese in the celery. Cut thin slivers of green pepper to place over cheese as garnish.

PEANUT BUTTER STUFFED CELERY

Blend equal parts peanut butter and whipped margarine or softened cream cheese; beat until light and fluffy. Use as filling for celery.

DEVILED HAM STUFFED CELERY

Blend together equal parts deviled ham spread and softened cream cheese to serve as stuffing for celery. Garnish with minced parsley or green pepper slivers.

TUNA-STUFFED CELERY

For the celery stuffing, drain and flake contents of chunk-style tuna, blend with a teaspoon of minced parsley, a tablespoon of minced onion (or a teaspoon of instant minced onion reconstituted with water), and just a little mayonnaise (1 to 2 tablespoons mayonnaise for 1 can tuna). Pile this lightly in trimmed celery stalks, sprinkle with paprika.

CHEESE DREAMS

Cut pieces of sliced American cheese to fit the tops of saltines. Place crackers on a baking sheet and slip under the broiler until cheese has started to melt. Eat while still warm.

PEANUT-CHEESE DREAMS

Spread saltines with peanut butter. Place slices of cheese cut to fit the saltines over the peanut butter. Place under broiler just until cheese starts to melt.

APPLEWICHES

Core apples, cut crosswise in thick slices. Put cheese slices between apples slices and eat like sandwiches.

CHEESE AND PINEAPPLE KABOBS

Chunks of cheese must be used for these, about 1-inch square. Put cheese and pineapple chunks or wedges alternately on extra-long cocktail picks, then roll in coconut or crushed nuts. This is party food, very good served with fruit punch.

POPSICLE CUBES

Use refrigerator freezing trays to make frozen goodies. Pour fruit juice (orange juice, pineapple juice, Hawaiian Punch, etc.) into the trays; in each divider, place fruit, such as maraschino cherries or drained crushed pineapple or chopped up canned peaches. When cubes are partially frozen, insert wooden flat sticks in ice. (These can be purchased in some hardware stores and variety stores.) When cubes are frozen solid (this will take at least 4 hours), remove from tray, serve like commercial Popsicles (to be sucked from the stick). (Fruit unless very small should be chopped, otherwise the solidly frozen fruit is hard to eat. *Crushed nuts or shredded coconut can also be added.*)

HAWAIIAN BANANA BITES

Cut peeled bananas into 1-inch lengths. Roll in shredded coconut. Or, roll in crushed peanuts. Very good with milk shakes.

CRACKER TOWERS

Piles of crackers can be spread with any soft cheese spread (pimiento, cheddar, bacon-flavored, chive cheese or Roquefort cream) in alternate layers, with about 4 crackers in each pile. Or, spread the crackers with peanut butter, mayonnaise, margarine, cream cheese with chopped nuts, or peanut butter and jam in alternate layers.

These are fun for youngsters to make themselves. Put out saltines and a selection of spreads. Cream cheese and peanut butter in alternate layers make a nice combination. Pimiento cheese spread is good with strawberry jam, too.

CARROT STICKS

Select small rather than large carrots; scrape and cut lengthwise into slivers. Soak slivers in salted ice water for half an hour; drain, pat dry with paper towel, wrap in small quantities in sandwich size plastic bags and seal with a tie-wrap to keep crisp in refrigerator. It's better to package them in small portions for once the bag is opened, the carrots lose some of their crispness.

(For other good afternoon or bedtime snacks, see *Fruited Gelatins, Puddings,* and *Cookies.*)

Sandwiches

Most American children insist on spongy white bread for their sandwiches, which is unfortunate, for this type of bread is much less nutritious than firmer whole-grain breads. Despite the claims of the commercial bakeries, such bread even when enriched with added riboflavin, niacin, thiamin and other vitamins, is less desirable than whole grain products. This is because the refining and bleaching process removes every bit of the bran, in which the greatest food values lie. Part of the vitamins and minerals are replaced, but a synthetic source of these food elements is never as good as a natural source.

For this reason it's important to start children as young as possible on whole wheat, cracked wheat, and other whole grain cereal products. Sandwiches made with these and with rye, pumpernickel, Boston brown bread, date-nut bread and Anadama (a cornmeal-rye combination) are much more nutritious than those made with the spongy sandwich loaves. The whole grain or unrefined flours actually have much more flavor, and if children learn while young to like such breads, you will already have gained a victory.

The unsliced whole wheat bread produced by Pepperidge Farms is much more flavorful than the same bread packaged and sold already sliced—commercial slicing does subtly but distinctly cause a loss of flavor. Unfortunately the unsliced loaf is less available in supermarkets, sometimes only on special order. It may be worthwhile shopping in health stores for breads made with whole grains, if your child's appetite is so poor there is reason to believe he is undernourished. Most children seem to like rye bread with sliced cheese, ham, or bologna. Both

Boston brown bread and date-nut bread are delicious with cream cheese or cottage cheese as a filling.

The Peanut Butter Family

Every American mother knows about peanut butter-and-jelly sandwiches. How is it possible to raise an American child otherwise? If the number of peanut butter-and-jelly sandwiches put together daily in American kitchens were laid end to end, they would probably reach from Boston Harbor to San Diego Bay (and maybe back again).

Peaunt butter is classed as a protein food, though not a complete protein and not sufficiently high in protein to qualify for one of the required "2 or more servings a day" of meat or meat substitutes.

Here are some other peanut butter combinations which may appeal to your persnickety youngster:

peanut butter + cottage cheese/on cracked wheat bread
peanut butter + cooked crumbled bacon/on whole wheat toast
peanut butter + grated carrots/on enriched white bread
peanut butter + cream cheese + tomato catsup/on white bread
peanut butter + margarine + thin-sliced ham or bologna/on rye bread
peanut butter + applesauce/on Boston brown bread

Tomato Sandwich Combinations

There are two drawbacks to tomato sandwiches: the tomatoes must be sliced and added to the sandwich just before eating—otherwise they weep, and even when freshly cut, they tend to squash into juice when clutched by little hands. But considering how much important food value tomato provides in the diet, these disadvantages should be taken in stride, especially in the summer when tomatoes are in season and inexpensive.

Here are some good combinations:

plain sliced tomatoes sprinkled with salt/on buttered white bread
sliced tomatoes + cream cheese/on whole wheat bread
sliced tomatoes + lettuce + mayonnaise/on white bread
tomatoes + crisp bacon/on toasted white or whole wheat bread
tomatoes + sliced American or Swiss cheese + mayonnaise + lettuce/on white, rye, or pumpernickel bread
tomatoes + sliced ham or bologna + mustard or mayonnaise/ on white or cracked wheat bread

Grilled Cheese Combinations

Children like to make these themselves, as soon as they are old enough to handle a skillet or electric sandwich grill. The safest and easiest way is to spread one piece of bread on one side with margarine, place that slice margarine-side down in a skillet, lay a slice of cheese on the bread, then spread a second bread slice with margarine and place that on the cheese margarine-side up. The heat can be turned on under the skillet (or the grill plugged in) *after* the sandwich is so put together. This eliminates danger of spattering from grease and there is less likelihood of fingers getting burned by touching the hot edge of skillet or grill.

If made in a sandwich grill, both sides of the sandwich will be toasted at once, no turning is necessary. If made in a skillet, the sandwich must be turned as soon as the bread on the bottom is golden.

White bread is the only suitable kind to use for grilled cheese sandwiches. Other kinds just don't seem to taste right.

GRILLED CHEESE AND HAM (OR BOLOGNA)

Place a thin slice of ham or bologna on top of the slice of cheese before adding second slice of bread.

GRILLED CHEESE AND TOMATO

Add one or two tomato slices to the cheese.

GRILLED SALAMI AND MOZZARELLA

Instead of American cheese, use thin slices of mozzarella cheese, cover this with thin slices of salami.

GRILLED CHEESE AND PICKLES

Add thinly sliced dill pickles to the cheese before adding second slice of bread.

Cottage Cheese Combinations

Cottage cheese + ham or bologna + mustard/on whole wheat or pumpernickel bread
Cottage cheese + peach jam/on Boston brown bread
Cottage cheese + bacon + sliced tomato/on whole wheat or pumpernickel
Cottage cheese + currant jelly/on date nut bread

Meat Sandwich Combinations

Sliced ham + Swiss or American cheese + mustard/on white or whole wheat bread
Sliced ham + cream cheese + watercress/on white or whole wheat bread

Sliced ham + sliced sweet gherkin pickles + butter or margarine/on cracked wheat bread

Bologna + potato salad/on cracked wheat, white or rye bread

Salami + cream cheese/on rye bread

Sliced roast beef + lettuce + mayonnaise/on white bread

Sliced meat loaf + mustard + mayonnaise or catsup/on white bread

Sliced chicken or turkey + lettuce + mayonnaise/on whole wheat bread

CHEESE-NUT SANDWICH

(3 to 5 Sandwiches)

1 3-oz. package cream cheese, softened
¼ cup finely chopped peanuts or walnuts
1 can Boston brown bread, or 1 small loaf date-nut bread

Cheese must be soft enough to spread easily. Add nuts, blend well. Slice the brown bread as thinly as possible; date-nut bread may be cut a little thicker. Spread cheese-nut mixture between bread slices. If made more than an hour in advance, refrigerate sandwiches until time to serve. (Number of sandwiches depends on how many slices can be obtained from bread and how thickly filling is spread.)

TUNA SALAD SANDWICH FILLING

(For 5 or 6 Sandwiches)

1 7-oz. can tuna, well-drained
½ cup minced celery
2 to 3 tablespoons mayonnaise
2 small gherkin pickles, chopped (optional)
Few drops lemon juice
Salt and pepper to taste

In a bowl combine tuna, celery, chopped pickles, and mayonnaise. Mix lightly with a fork. Add lemon juice, salt and pepper from shakers; taste to determine whether it's seasoned enough.

This can be stored in a bowl in the refrigerator, covered with plastic wrap, until needed.

Young children like to make their own tuna salad sandwiches—it's one of the first things they learn to do in the kitchen. With adult supervision, the celery can be chopped in an electric blender; or, use only gherkin pickles (which are far easier for little fingers to cut with a paring knife) and omit the celery.

Serve between slices of whole wheat or cracked wheat bread, with or without lettuce and mayonnaise.

EGG SALAD SANDWICH FILLING

(For 5 or 6 Sandwiches)

4 hard-cooked eggs, shelled
½ cup minced celery
1 teaspoon minced parsley (optional)
2 to 3 tablespoons mayonnaise
¼ teaspoon prepared mustard (optional)

Chop eggs in a blender or on a board with paring knife. Cut celery in the blender. Combine eggs, celery, and remaining ingredients, blend lightly with fork. Good between buttered whole heat, rye, pumpernickel or Boston brown bread.

CHICKEN SALAD SANDWICH FILLING

1 cup diced cooked chicken
¼ cup minced celery
2 to 3 tablespoons mayonnaise
1 teaspoon catsup (optional)
Salt, pepper

Combine ingredients; use as filling for sandwiches made with white, whole wheat or cracked wheat bread.

HAM SALAD SANDWICH FILLING

Prepare as for Chicken Salad, substituting 1 cup diced cooked ham for the chicken, and using prepared mustard in place of catsup.

ROAST BEEF SALAD SANDWICH FILLING

Prepare as for Chicken Salad, substituting 1 cup minced cooked leftover roast beef for the chicken, and mustard or horseradish in place of or in addition to the catsup.

Other sandwich fillings can also be made with chopped cooked tongue, luncheon meat, leftover roast pork, or leftover pot roast.

For picnics or any outdoor meals, place the salad sandwich filling in hot dog buns instead of between slices of bread—much easier to eat, with less danger of the salad spilling out.

Pizzas

Frozen pizzas, ready to thrust into the oven, are acceptable to most youngsters, and most American mothers with ample freezer space will probably resort to these. But pizzas made with packaged mix are also very easy to prepare, as are those made from hot roll mix. And when an individual pizza is demanded, a substitute that's not bad can be made with refrigerated ready-to-bake biscuits or rolls pressed flat, or with English muffins. Or even with corn muffins!

Making pizza dough from scratch is not hard, and those children who enjoy cooking may want to learn to make their own.

CORN MUFFIN PIZZAS

Use the packaged corn muffins or corn toasties (the kind that can be slipped into a toaster). For each serving, place mozzarella or Swiss cheese on the corn muffin, cover cheese with tomato sauce, and top with crumbled cooked bacon. Sprinkle with oregano, minced parsley, salt and pepper. Bake in oven preheated to 400°F until cheese is melted, about 6 minutes.

PIZZA DOUGH

(Makes 2 Pizzas)

1 envelope active dry yeast
1 cup warm (not hot) water
1 teaspoon salt
4 tablespoons olive oil
3½ cups sifted all-purpose unbleached flour
½ teaspoon sugar (optional)

Sprinkle yeast over warm water in a large mixing bowl. Stir in salt and 2 tablespoons of the olive oil, then add flour mixed with sugar a little at a time, until all has been added. Beat with a spoon until smooth, then lift up dough and turn out onto a lightly floured board and knead with fingers (punching, pressing, and rolling) until dough is elastic. Replace dough in the bowl, brush a little oil over the top, cover the bowl lightly with waxed paper, and let rise in a warm place free from drafts until dough is doubled in bulk. Then cut the dough into halves with a knife, remove one half at a time, roll into a ball, and press the dough with the "heel" of the palm to fit a 14-inch pizza pan or baking sheet, making the dough slightly thicker and higher around the edges. Do the same with the second ball of dough. Brush both with additional olive oil, then add the tomato sauce and other desired ingredients. If only one pizza is wanted now, freeze the second one for later baking.

Bake filled pizza in oven preheated to 450°F for 20 to 25 minutes or until crust is golden.

For extra nutrition, add ⅓ cup instant nonfat dry milk to the flour when preparing the pizza dough.

To freeze pizzas: Place shaped, filled dough in pan in freezer until firm, then remove from pan and cover with plastic wrap, sealing edges. To bake frozen pizza, remove plastic wrap, place in oven directly on the rack without defrosting; bake until dough is golden.

SAUSAGE-GRINDER PIZZA

1 pizza crust, unbaked
1 tablespoon olive oil
¼ pound Italian sweet sausage, cut in small pieces
½ green pepper, cut in strips
1 canned pimiento, cut in strips
1 small onion, sliced
1 cup tomato sauce
¼ cup Parmesan cheese

Fit dough into pizza pan or baking sheet. In a skillet, saute sausage, green pepper, pimiento and onion in olive oil until vegetables are tender. Spoon this over the pizza dough. Cover with tomato sauce and the cheese. Bake in oven preheated to 450°F for 20 to 25 minutes until crust is golden.

Note: This may be frozen to be baked later. If baked when still frozen, just add an extra 5 to 10 minutes to baking time.

CHEESE-TOPPED PIZZA

1 pizza crust, unbaked
1 8-oz. can tomato sauce
¼ teaspoon oregano
1 teaspoon minced parsley
½ teaspoon instant minced onion
2 tablespoons olive oil
1 large tomato, peeled and sliced
Salt, pepper
4 or 5 slices mozzarella cheese, sliced thin
¼ cup grated Parmesan cheese

Shape pizza dough in pan or on baking sheet. In a saucepan, combine the tomato sauce, oregano, parsley, onion, garlic and olive oil. Simmer 5 minutes. Place sliced tomatoes over the dough; sprinkle tomato slices with salt and pepper from shakers. Place slices of mozzarella over the tomatoes. Pour the tomato sauce over the tomatoes and cheese. Top with grated Parmesan. Bake in oven preheated to 450°F for 20 to 25 minutes.

CHEESE PIZZA DOUGH

½ recipe Pizza Dough
½ cup shredded Cheddar cheese

While kneading pizza dough (made according to recipe on page 67), work the cheese into it with fingers. After the dough has risen, and is ready to roll out, fit it into a 14-inch pizza pan or baking sheet. Top it with any of the usual pizza fillings, or with the following:

3 large tomatoes, sliced
Salt, pepper
¼ teaspoon oregano
4 slices bacon, cooked, crumbled
1 teaspoon minced parsley
½ cup Parmesan cheese

Lay tomatoes over pizza dough in overlapping slices. Sprinkle with salt, pepper, and oregano. Sprinkle bacon and parsley over tomato slices and finally the chese. Bake in oven preheated to 450°F for 20 to 25 minutes.

SLOPPY JOE PIZZA

1 pizza crust, unbaked
½ pound ground beef
1 tablespoon olive oil
½ teaspoon salt
Dash of pepper
½ cup chopped or sliced onion
1 garlic clove, minced
½ green pepper, chopped
1 8-oz. can tomato sauce
¼ cup grated Parmesan cheese

Fit unbaked pizza dough into 14-inch pizza pan or baking sheet. In skillet, sauté the beef in olive oil until it has lost its pink color; add salt, pepper, onion, garlic, and green pepper. Continue cooking until onions are soft. Add tomato sauce, simmer 2 or 3 minutes. Spread over pizza dough. Sprinkle Parmesan cheese over top. Bake in oven preheated to 450°F for 20 to 25 minutes until crust is golden.

Note: This or any other pizza filling can be used with packaged pizza mix or hot roll mix, following package directions. If pizza mix is used, the 10-oz. can of tomato sauce that comes with the mix may be used instead of the standard 8-oz. can of tomato sauce.

INDIVIDUAL BISCUIT PIZZAS

(Makes 10 Servings)

1 package refrigerated oven-ready biscuits or Parker House rolls
Mozzarella cheese or Swiss cheese
1 8-oz. can tomato sauce
Dash of oregano
Dash of garlic powder or garlic salt

Separate the biscuits or rolls, after opening the package according to directions. Press each biscuit or roll with fingers into a flat shape with raised edge. Place on baking sheet. On each place a slice of cheese, cut so that it does not reach to edge of pizzas. Spoon tomato sauce over the cheese. Sprinkle sauce with oregano and garlic powder or salt. Bake in oven preheated to 400°F for 8 to 10 minutes until the dough is golden.

Pancakes, Muffins, Other Quick Breads

The first cooking lesson for many young children is making Animal Pancakes. In the beginning, the batter is mixed by mother, but since making pancake batter with mix is as simple as any cooking operation can be, it needn't be long until the little ones start beating or shaking the batter themselves.

Pancakes can be served for lunch or supper as well as breakfast, filled with cottage cheese, or creamed tuna, or even leftover chicken warmed up in leftover chicken gravy. The pancakes themselves can be enriched with instant nonfat dry milk worked into the batter. The same is true of most other quick breads. And, as observed earlier in this book, using whole grain flour products instead of white flour is an important way of adding extra Vitamin B to the diet.

ANIMAL PANCAKES

To make the batter, use pancake mix or biscuit mix, following package directions. For extra nutrition, add ⅓ cup nonfat dry milk to the standard recipe calling for 2 cups mix.

To bake the pancakes, use an electric griddle or electric skillet set at 400°F (or if using a castiron griddle, heat until a drop of water dropped on the griddle evaporates instantly). It may be advisable to brush a small amount of fat over the surface of the griddle or skillet before the first pancakes are added—no more than a teaspoonful, well-distributed. The batter should be in a bowl rather than a pitcher; the child puts the batter on the griddle by spoonfuls, sometimes deliberately dribbling for effect. (Very tiny pancakes are "fairy pancakes" suitable for "feeding" to dolls—or to hungry-looking dogs.) Just what kind of animal will result is not always certain. To make a *cat* (the most popular), you drop one spoonful of batter on the griddle for the body, another smaller spoonful for the head, then let batter dribble from the body to form a tail.

A *turtle* is made by adding four tiny pancakes (the legs) around the perimeter of one round pancake about 3 inches in diameter.

Birds may end up looking more like *dragons*, and vice versa. It doesn't really matter what the pancake looks like. If having created his own images on a griddle gives an edge to the finicky child's breakfast appetite, the effort is worthwhile. Arrange the "animals" on a platter, dribble blended melted butter and syrup over the top.

HONEY BUNS

(8 Buns)

2 cups biscuit mix
1 egg
⅓ cup milk
2 tablespoons firm butter
¼ cup honey
2 tablespoons melted butter
⅓ cup brown sugar
⅓ cup chopped nuts (walnuts or almonds)
⅓ cup raisins
2 tablespoons additional honey

Combine biscuit mix, egg, and milk, beat with fork until sticky. Flour fingers, then knead biscuit dough until it can be handled easily. Roll out on floured board to a rectangle about 14x10 inches. Dot dough with bits of butter. Combine ¼ cup honey with melted butter and brown sugar, spread over dough; add chopped nuts and raisins. Roll up. Cut with knife into 8 slices. Place on greased baking sheet or baking pan close together. Spread additional honey over top. Bake in oven preheated to 400°F for 20 minutes or until golden.

CHEESE BISCUITS

(10 to 12 Biscuits)

2 cups biscuit mix
½ cup grated American or Cheddar cheese
⅔ cup milk

Combine all ingredients, stir with fork into soft dough, then beat until sticky. Knead with well-floured fingers into a ball, then roll out on floured board or press out with "heel" of palm directly onto ungreased baking sheet to ½-inch thick. Cut with floured biscuit cutter (in circles) or floured knife (in squares). Bake in oven preheated to 450°F until biscuits are golden and puffed, about 10 minutes.

FLANNEL CAKES

2 cups pancake or biscuit mix
1 egg
1½ cups buttermilk
Pinch of baking soda

Combine all ingredients, beat or shake until smooth. Let stand for 15 minutes, then bake on preheated skillet or griddle (400°F). These will be thick and spongy. Serve topped with syrup and butter. Serves 3 adults, or 2 adults and 2 children.

JOHNNY CAKES

(4 Family Servings)

1 package corn muffin mix
1 or 2 eggs
2 cups milk *

Combine all ingredients. Let stand 10 minutes. Bake on griddle or skillet set at 400°F as for regular pancakes. Serve with maple syrup and butter, accompanied by bacon or sausages.

* Buttermilk may be used instead of sweet milk; add a pinch of baking soda to the batter.

BRAN MUFFINS

(Makes 12)

1 cup sifted all-purpose unbleached flour
½ teaspoon salt
3 teaspoons baking powder
1 cup whole bran cereal
1 cup milk
2 tablespoons soft shortening or vegetable oil
¼ cup granulated sugar
1 egg

Grease 2 6-cup muffin pans. Combine sifted flour, salt, baking powder; blend well. Soak bran in milk about 5 minutes. Beat together soft shortening and egg; add bran and milk. Stir in flour mixture, only until dry ingredients are moistened. Fill muffin cups ⅔ full. Bake in oven preheated to 400°F for 20 to 25 minutes or until nicely browned.

CHEESE BLINTZES

(6 Family Servings)

1 cup biscuit or pancake mix
1 egg
1¼ cups milk
2 to 3 tablespoons butter
1 cup creamed cottage cheese
Sour cream

Make a batter of biscuit or pancake mix, egg and milk; beat until foamy (if you have an electric blender, place all ingredients in blender, beat 10 seconds). Make the pancakes in a small skillet (6- or 7-inches in diameter), adding 1 tablespoon batter at a time to hot skillet in which just enough butter has been melted to moisten surface. Roll skillet so thin batter will be evenly distributed. When golden on the bottom, flip with a spatula, cook until golden on the other side. When all batter has been cooked, fill pancakes with cottage cheese, using 2 tablespoons cottage cheese for each pancake. Roll up, place overlapped side down in a shallow casserole. Melt remaining butter and spoon over top. If dinner is delayed, keep pancakes warm in oven set at 200°F until time to serve. Serve topped with sour cream.

QUICK NUT-FRUIT BUNS

(Makes 10)

1 package refrigerated oven-ready dinner rolls (butterflake type)
½ cup raisins
½ cup chopped almonds or walnuts
Cinnamon-sugar mixture

Open package and separate rolls according to package directions. Set oven at 450°F. While oven is heating, push raisins and nuts down into the folds of the rolls. Sprinkle cinnamon-sugar mixture over top. Bake as directed until golden. Very nice for breakfast, or to serve with scrambled eggs for supper.

PINEAPPLE CORN MUFFINS

(Makes 12)

1 package corn muffin mix
2 eggs
½ cup crushed pineapple, including juice

Combine all ingredients in a mixing bowl, stir just until all dry ingredients are moistened. Grease 2 6-cup muffin tins; or, fill muffin tins with paper liners. Distribute batter in the cups, filling each half full. Bake in oven preheated to 375°F for 18 minutes until firm and golden.

BROWN FRUIT BREAD

¾ cup sifted all-purpose flour
1 teaspoon salt
1 teaspoon baking soda
1 cup unsifted whole wheat flour
1 tablespoon softened margarine
½ cup brown sugar
1 egg
1 tablespoon grated orange peel
1 cup milk
¼ cup vinegar
1 tablespoon orange juice
½ cup chopped nuts
⅔ cup seedless raisins

You will need 2 empty food cans to use as "pans" for this bread: 1-lb. tomato cans are fine. If tops have been removed by an electric can-opener, leaving smooth edges, they should be as easy to use as any other baking utensils. Grease insides generously. Preheat oven to 350°F. Sift all-purpose flour, salt and soda together; stir in whole wheat flour. In electric mixer or blender, beat together the margarine, sugar, egg, and orange peel until smooth; add milk, vinegar and orange juice, then add flour mixture a little at a time, beating continuously until well-blended. Finally add nuts and raisins, stirring to distribute well throughout batter. Pour batter into cans; fit aluminum foil or buttered brown paper over top of cans, tie on top with butcher's cord. Bake 1 hour and 15 minutes. Remove from oven, cool 5 minutes on rack, then run knife around edges to loosen bread. Cut in horizontal slices to serve.

GRAHAM GEMS

(Makes 12)

¾ cup all-purpose unbleached flour
4 teaspoons baking powder
½ teaspoon salt
¼ cup white or brown sugar
1 cup unsifted whole wheat flour
1 egg
1 cup milk
¼ cup vegetable oil

Sift together all-purpose flour, baking powder, salt and sugar. Stir in whole wheat flour. Form a well in center of flour mixture. Add egg, milk, and salad oil, beat just until dry ingredients are thoroughly moistened. Grease 2 6-cup muffin tins. Spoon batter into cups, filling ⅔ full. Wipe off any batter that dribbles on edges. Bake in oven preheated to 375°F until muffins are evenly browned, about 35 minutes. Let muffins cool in pans about 5 minutes, then loosen by running knife around edge—they should slip out easily. Serve hot with plenty of butter.

Egg and Cheese Dishes

FRENCH TOAST FOR ONE

1 egg yolk
2 tablespoons milk
1 teaspoon sugar (optional)
1 slice white bread
1 tablespoon bacon fat or butter

Beat together egg yolk and milk, stir in sugar. Soak bread in mixture, turning once so that it will be moistened on each side. Melt bacon drippings or margarine in a small skillet; when hot, add soaked bread, sauté until golden on each side. Serve with syrup.

FRENCH TOAST FOR TWO

1 egg
¼ cup milk
2 teaspoons sugar
2 to 3 slices white bread
1 to 2 tablespoons bacon fat or butter

Beat together egg, milk and sugar. Soak bread in mixture 1 slice at a time; sauté in hot fat until golden on each side. Serve with syrup.

FRIED EGG ON TOAST

The egg is not really fried: it is steamed in butter. The butter is melted in a small skillet over low heat, then, as soon as it is melted, before it sizzles, an egg is broken into the butter carefully, so the yolk does not break. Sprinkle salt over the egg very lightly, place a cover over the pan, cook just until egg white is firm but yolk still soft. Meantime make toast (whole wheat toast, preferably), and butter it while hot. Slip the egg out of the skillet very carefully, using a pancake turner, taking care that the soft yolk does not break. Put the egg over the toast. When the yolk is broken, it will run into the toast like a sauce.

BAKED CHEESE FONDUE

(6 Family Servings)

6 to 8 slices white bread, crusts trimmed
1 cup grated sharp Cheddar cheese
3 eggs, beaten
4 cups milk
½ teaspoon prepared mustard
¼ teaspoon salt
Dash of pepper

Butter a 1½-quart casserole. Place bread in casserole, cutting to fit in flat layers. Spread cheese between each layer. Combine eggs, milk, mustard, salt and pepper; pour mixture over the bread. Let soak 1 hour. Preheat oven to 350°F. Bake 45 minutes or until top is puffy and golden.

SHIRRED EGGS

For each serving, you need an individual ramekin or casserole. Place a teaspoon of butter in each; place in oven set at 400°F just until butter is melted. Break an egg into each ramekin (for larger ramekins, 2 eggs may be added); sprinkle eggs with salt and pepper from shakers. Add 1 tablespoon milk to each ramekin. Place in oven at 375°F just until eggs are set, about 5 minutes for single eggs, 10 minutes if 2 eggs are baked in each ramekin.

SOUFFLÉD FRENCH TOAST

(2 Servings)

2 eggs, separated
¼ cup milk
Salt, pepper
1 teaspoon sugar
2 to 3 slices white bread
1 tablespoon butter
1 tablespoon oil

Combine egg yolks and milk, salt, pepper, and sugar. Beat egg whites until stiff; fold into yolk mixture. Pour this over bread slices; turn once. Heat butter and oil until sizzling; lower heat, add bread and sauté until puffed and golden on each side. Serve with a tart jam.

CHEESE MILK TOAST

(1 Serving)

2 slices enriched white or whole wheat bread
Butter or margarine
¼ cup shredded Swiss or American cheese
1 cup steaming hot milk
Salt, pepper

Toast the bread; while hot spread with butter or margarine. Place in soup plate or bowl. Spread cheese over the toast. Add hot milk. Sprinkle with salt and pepper from shakers.

Note: For a finicky eater, this may be too much for 1 serving. In that case use only 1 slice of bread, omit cheese or use only 1 tablespoon, and add ½ cup hot milk.

SCRAMBLED EGGS AND FRANKFURTERS

(2 Servings)

2 frankfurters, cut in ¼-inch slices
2 tablespoons butter
3 eggs, beaten
¼ teaspoon salt
2 tablespoons milk

Saute the frankfurter slices in butter until lightly browned. Stir salt and milk into eggs, add mixture to pan; lift with spatula as egg firms until firm throughout but still moist. Serve for breakfast or supper.

COTTAGE CHEESE SOUFFLÉ

(3 Servings)

1 cup cottage cheese
2 tablespoons butter or chicken fat, melted
2 eggs, separated
3 tablespoons light cream or homogenized milk
½ teaspoon salt
Dash of pepper
2 tablespoons blanched shredded almonds

Combine cottage cheese with melted butter or chicken fat, the egg yolks, cream, salt and pepper. Blend well. Separately beat egg whites until stiff; fold into cottage cheese mixture with the nuts. Spoon into greased 1-quart casserole. Bake in oven preheated to 350°F for 20 to 25 minutes until golden on top. Serve immediately as an entree with spinach or other green vegetable.

EGGS FLAMENCO

(4 Servings)

The same as SHIRRED EGGS (page 77) except that the eggs bake in tomato sauce:

1 8-ounce can tomato sauce
1 teaspoon instant minced onion
2 tablespoons olive oil or salad oil
1 teaspoon minced parsley
4 eggs
Salt, pepper
Grated Parmesan cheese (optional)

Combine tomato sauce with onion, oil, and parsley. Divide among 4 ramekins. Break an egg into each. Sprinkle salt and pepper from shakers over the eggs; sprinkle cheese over top. Bake in oven preheated to 400°F just until whites of eggs have set, 8 to 12 minutes.

SKILLET EGGS AND CHEESE

(4 Servings)

2 tablespoons butter
4 very thin slices Swiss or Provolone cheese
4 eggs
Salt, pepper

Melt butter in 10-inch skillet. Place slices of cheese in the butter; lower heat. Break eggs over the cheese. Sprinkle with salt and pepper. Cover skillet; cook just until whites of eggs are set. Carefully cut the eggs and cheese to separate, then remove from pan one by one with pancake turner. Serve on or with toast.

BUNNY EGGS

(Eggs and Tomatoes in Buns)

(4 Servings)

4 hamburger buns
4 slices tomato
3 to 4 teaspoons sugar
Salt, pepper
1 teaspoon instant minced onion
4 eggs
Grated cheese

Use buns that are not pre-sliced; cut a slice from top, scoop out centers, leaving a hollow. Fit a tomato slice into each hollow, sprinkle tomato with sugar, salt and pepper and minced onion. Break an egg over each tomato slice; sprinkle the eggs with salt, pepper, and cheese. Bake in oven preheated to 375°F until eggs are set and cheese melted or lightly browned.

CHEESE WESTERN

(3 or 4 Servings)

1 small onion, minced or thinly sliced
½ green pepper, diced (optional)
1 tomato, chopped
2 tablespoons olive or salad oil
½ teaspoon salt
4 eggs, beaten
Toast

Saute the onion, green pepper, and tomato in oil until soft and lightly browned. (If green pepper does not meet with the finicky one's taste, omit it.) Sprinkle salt over the vegetables as they cook. Pour in beaten eggs, lifting up and over with a spatula. Serve immediately on toast, or between slices of toast as a sandwich.

CREAMED EGGS

(3 to 6 Servings)

- 6 hard-cooked eggs, quartered
- 3 tablespoons butter or margarine
- 1 tablespoon minced scallions or onion
- 3 tablespoons flour
- ½ teaspoon salt
- Dash of pepper
- 2 cups milk
- Dash of nutmeg or curry powder (optional)

Melt butter in skillet or saucepan; add scallions or onion, cook until soft. Stir in flour, cook until it bubbles. Add salt and pepper and slowly stir in milk, cooking over low heat until smooth and thickened. Season as desired. Add eggs, keep over heat just until eggs are heated through. Serve over toast. For a heartier entree, serve accompanied by crisp cooked bacon. Number of servings depends on age, appetites, and fiinickiness of children and adults being served.

Sauce hint: If you have a blender, place all ingredients but eggs in it, beat until mixture is smooth, then pour into saucepan and stir over low heat until sauce is bubbly and thickened.

CREAMED EGGS AND HAM

Exactly like CREAMED EGGS AND CHICKEN (page 83) except that minced or chopped leftover baked ham is used in place of chicken and condensed cream of celery or mushroom soup may be used in place of cream of chicken soup.

EGGS BAKED IN NESTS

(6 Servings)

6 slices very soft white bread
Margarine
6 eggs
Salt, pepper
Grated Cheddar or Parmesan cheese (optional)

Preheat oven to 400°F. Fit bread slices into cups of a 6-cup muffin tin, pushing down to form a "nest" (the spongy type of bread is best for this). Spread margarine on bread. Place in oven until bread is very lightly toasted. Remove, break an egg into each nest. Sprinkle eggs with salt, pepper, and cheese. Return to oven and bake until whites are set and yolks firm, about 20 minutes. Slip "nests" from muffin tins carefully. After they have cooled just a little, these can be picked up and eaten with fingers. They are good for breakfast, lunch, snacks, or supper.

POTATO OMELET

(2 Servings)

1 small potato, peeled, minced
2 tablespoons minced onion
2 to 3 tablespoons olive oil
½ teaspoon salt
3 eggs, beaten

The quickest way to mince the potatoes and onion is in an electric blender. Follow manufacturer's instructions. Or, chop on a chopping board with a wide-bladed French knife. Add vegetables to oil in skillet; cook until soft and lightly browned. Sprinkle vegetables with salt as they cook. When potatoes are tender, add beaten egg, lifting up edges with a spatula as the egg firms to allow moist egg to run under. When omelet is golden on bottom, place 5 inches from heat in broiler oven until top is lightly browned. Cut in pie-shaped wedges to serve. Hearty, a meal in itself, the omelet may be accompanied by sliced tomatoes or cole slaw and hot rolls.

(Instead of mincing potato and onion, both may be thinly-sliced. The important thing is that both vegetables must be thoroughly cooked before egg is added.)

CREAMED EGGS AND CHICKEN

(3 Adult or 6 Child Servings)

1 10-oz. can condensed cream of chicken soup
⅓ cup homogenized milk, or half-and-half, or evaporated milk
Pinch of curry powder (optional)
1 cup cut-up cooked or canned chicken, or leftover roast turkey
6 hard-cooked eggs, quartered
Minced parsley

Combine soup and milk or half-and-half; heat until it bubbles. Season with curry powder. Add eggs, chicken and parsley. Serve with cooked rice.

TUNA OMELET

(4 Family Servings)

1 7-oz. can tuna fish, drained
1 small onion, thinly sliced
2 tablespoons chopped green pepper; or 1 tablespoon minced parsley
1 tablespoon butter
1 small tomato, chopped
½ teaspoon salt
4 eggs, beaten

Break up drained tuna with fork. Sauté onion and green pepper (or parsley) in butter until soft. Add tomato; cook until very soft. Add tuna. Sprinkle salt over mixture. Pour in half of beaten eggs, lifting up edges with spatula and tilting pan so liquid egg can run under. When first part of egg is firm, add remaining egg; lifting as before. When omelet is golden on bottom, place in preheated broiler oven 5 inches from heat just until lightly browned on top. Cut in wedges to serve.

Soups

Most parents take the easy way out and rely on canned or dehydrated soups most of the time, and as far as most children are concerned, this is fine with them. So, most of the following suggestions are tricks to make canned or dehydrated soups either more appealing or to give them added nutrition.

A few soups "made from scratch" are included because I have found these to be great hits with children and adults alike and they are, in addition, quite easy to prepare.

CREAM OF TOMATO SOUP

This is one of the most popular of soups with children, and it is bursting with nutrition. The canned condensed tomato soup pleases nearly everyone (but gourmets), but here are a few tips to make it still more appealing:

• Always add *cold milk* to the soup concentrate, and stir it in a little at a time. Otherwise, the milk may curdle. Or, if you have a blender, it's safe to dump milk and tomato soup concentrate into the blender simultaneously, spin until the two are thoroughly blended, then warm in a saucepan over moderate heat, stirring constantly.

• For added nutrition, add ⅓ cup instant nonfat dry milk to the mixture of whole milk and condensed soup.

• Another way to add nutrition: sprinkle grated cheese (Cheddar or Parmesan) over the hot soup at table.

• Snipped parsley added to the soup gives it more attractive color and adds food value. (Fresh parsley is rich in vitamins A, B, and C and also a good source of iron.) Use parsley generously—a teaspoon of it to each serving is not too much.

• Crisp croutons are good with tomato soup, too. Cut stale white bread in cubes the size of poker dice, toast in the oven

(350°F) until delicately golden, about 5 minutes. Serve this way or toss with melted butter or margarine before adding to the soup.

• Make it a *Floating Island Soup:* Separate 2 eggs, beat the whites until stiff, then add the egg yolks to the milk and soup concentrate in a blender, beat until smooth. Warm soup slowly over moderate heat, stirring constantly, until heated through. Do *not* allow to boil. Drop spoonfuls of the beaten egg white over servings of the hot soup to form "islands." This will delight younger children and give them three of nature's most healthful foods in one dish.

CHICKEN NOODLE VEGETABLE SOUP

(4 Servings)

A good way to slip vegetables into a favorite food.

2 tablespoons butter
2 to 3 tablespoons chopped onion
1 small carrot, scraped, grated
¼ cup minced celery
1 to 2 teaspoons minced parsley
1 10-oz. can condensed chicken noodle soup
1 soup can of water

Melt the butter in a saucepan (do not allow it to brown). Add the vegetables and parsley, cook over moderate heat until onion is soft, then add canned soup and water and cook 5 minutes longer.

INSTANT MINESTRONE

(4 to 6 Child Servings)

Combine in a large saucepan 1 can condensed vegetable soup, 1 can condensed chicken noodle soup, 1 soup can of water, 1 cup canned white or kidney beans, well-drained, and 2 or 3 tablespoons minced parsley. Bring to a boil, simmer 3 or 4 minutes until heated through, then serve topped with grated Parmesan cheese.

CHICKEN NOODLE SOUP

Another child favorite, good just as it comes from the can, diluted with water. Or dress it up in any of these ways:

• Sprinkle snipped parsley over the soup as it is heating. (See comments on health value of parsley on page 84.)

• Let child help himself to grated cheese as a topping.

• If you happen to have any bits of leftover chicken or turkey in the refrigerator, even the last scrapings from a carcass, mince it up and add to the soup. Or, add minced cooked pork (leftover from roast or chops).

• Minced hard-cooked egg also makes a colorful, tasty and nutritious garnish.

TOMATO-CHICKEN-RICE SOUP

(4 Servings)

Combine 1 10-oz. can chicken with rice soup and 1 soup can of tomato juice in a saucepan; add paper-thin slices of carrot or celery to the soup. Heat to boiling, lower heat, simmer 3 or 4 minutes.

LENTIL SOUP

(6 to 8 Servings)

1 large onion, chopped
1 green pepper, seeded, diced
4 carrots, scraped, diced fine
4 tablespoons olive oil or butter
1 1-lb. can tomatoes
1 tablespoon salt
1 lb. lentils
8 cups water

Place onion, pepper and carrots in a large kettle with the oil or butter. Cook over moderate heat until vegetables are soft. Add remaining ingredients (lentils need not be previously soaked). Bring slowly to a boil, turn heat very low, simmer covered for 2 hours or until lentils are tender. If much water evaporates, add more as needed. This may be served plain, or topped with shredded Swiss cheese or grated Parmesan. It's a soup which my finicky child has always loved, and most other children seem to take to it, too.

Added attractions: it costs only pennies, and tastes even better when reheated.

TUNA CHOWDER

(6 to 8 Servings)

2½ cups milk
1 can cream of celery or cream of mushroom soup
1 can New England style clam chowder
1 7-oz. can tuna fish, well-drained and flaked
1 tablespoon minced parsley; or 1 hard-cooked egg, minced

If you have a blender, put 1 cup of milk in blender with the 2 soups, beat until smooth. (If you don't have a blender, place soups first in saucepan, stir in milk, then add tuna.) Transfer mixture from blender to saucepan, add remaining milk and the tuna, simmer, stirring, 10 minutes or until thoroughly heated. Serve garnished with parsely or egg. This is hearty, a good family entree for supper.

CORN-AND-BACON CHOWDER

(6 Family Servings)

2 tablespoons butter or margarine
1 tablespoon flour
1 1-lb. can cream-style corn
1 cup diced cooked potatoes or mashed potatoes
1 tablespoon instant minced onion
1 quart milk
Salt to taste
Dash of paprika
6 slices bacon, cooked, crumbled

Melt butter in deep saucepan or kettle. Stir in flour, cook until it bubbles. Add all remaining ingredients but bacon. (Leftover potatoes may be used, or use mashed potatoes made from mix.) Simmer 10 to 15 minutes. Sprinkle crumbled bacon over top of each serving.

SPLIT PEA WITH FRANKFURTERS

(6 to 8 Family Servings)

1 cup split peas (yellow or green)
3 quarts water
1 ham bone
1 small onion, chopped or sliced
2 sprigs celery leaves
4 sprigs parsley
Pinch of thyme
2 teaspoons salt, or to taste
Freshly ground black pepper
2 cups milk; or ⅔ cup instant nonfat dry milk and 1½ cups water
3 frankfurters, sliced
Toasted croutons (optional)

Soak split peas in water to cover overnight (unless they are the quick-cooking type which do not require soaking). Drain well. Add 3 quarts fresh water to peas in a large kettle, along with ham bone, onion, celery, parsley sprigs and thyme; add pepper. Bring to a boil, simmer, covered, over lowest heat for 2 hours or until peas are tender. Stir occasionally to prevent sticking. When peas are soft, remove bone, force soup through sieve. Add milk slowly; reheat, stirring. Add sliced frankfurters. Simmer until frankfurters are heated through. Serve this way or topped with croutons. This, too, is a soup nearly all children like—and the freshly made split pea soup is far better than that from a can or made with dehydrated mix.

Hamburgers, Hot Dogs, and Other Meat Dishes

You may grow bored with hamburgers five times a week, but children seldom do. And when you have prepared a gourmet company meat dish which your finicky one greets with a sneer, for heaven's sake don't waste such good food on his undeveloped palate. Throw him a hamburger or a hot dog and save wear and tear on your culinary pride.

I've found the best way to keep meat ground for hamburgers in readiness for emergencies is to buy it in quantity, then subdivide the meat into portions enough for 2 or 3 hamburgers. These portions I wrap separately in plastic bags and store in the freezer. In such portions, the chopped meat will defrost in the refrigerator in about 6 hours. Take it out of the freezer in the morning and by suppertime it will be ready to form into patties.

Ground chuck is the best and most economical beef cut to use for hamburgers. The meat sold in supermarkets as "hamburger meat" contains considerably more fat (and sometimes water) and the patties will shrink down in cooking to about half the size of those made with chuck.

As for "hot dogs," frankfurters, too, can be kept in the freezer wrapped in meal-size portions. I keep on hand some packets containing only 2 frankfurters, some containing 4, some 6. In this way, it is easy to cook enough for just one child, or for 2 or 3 children, as needed. In a large family, this may not be necessary since frankfurters will keep fresh in the refrigerator for a week, sometimes longer, but if not used within ten days, they tend to start forming a slime on the outside—and are not safe to use.

Frozen frankfurters can go directly from freezer to boiling hot water without defrosting.

The buns for both hamburgers and hot dogs can be kept in the freezer, too; if kept in bread box or refrigerator they turn stale all too quickly. To defrost quickly, stick the frozen buns in the oven set at 300°F; as soon as soft enough, open so that inside will defrost. This takes about 4 minutes.

ENRICHED HAMBURGERS

(2 Servings)

- ½ lb. ground chuck
- ¼ cup instant nonfat dry milk
- ½ teaspoon salt
- 1 teaspoon instant minced onion, reconstituted (optional)
- 1 teaspoon oil, butter or margarine

Combine beef, milk, salt, and onion (softened in water), mixing with fingers with a light motion until well-blended but still fluffy. Form into 2 plump patties. Saute in oil or butter until well-browned on each side. (If using a Teflon-coated skillet, the oil or butter may be omitted.) Serve in toasted hamburger buns, with the usual selection of relishes: catsup, piccalilli, mustard, sliced onions, India relish, etc.

EXTRA JUICY HAMBURGERS

(4 to 6 Servings)

- 1 lb. ground chuck
- 1 egg, beaten
- ½ cup crushed crackers
- ⅓ cup instant nonfat dry milk
- ¼ cup catsup
- ¾ teaspoon salt
- 1 teaspoon oil or bacon fat

Combine all ingredients but oil or fat; work with fingers until well-blended. Form into 4 or 6 hamburger patties. Heat oil or fat in skillet until it sizzles; place patties in skillet, turn heat low and sauté slowly until well-browned on each side, about 15 minutes. These will be softer in texture and juicier than burgers cooked quickly over high heat.

BURGERS AND ONIONS

Slice 1 large onion; fry it in 2 tablespoons bacon fat or butter until lightly browned. Serve as a relish over hamburgers in buns—this is enough for 4 hamburgers.

SLOPPY JOES

(6 Servings)

1 tablespoon bacon fat
1 lb. hamburger meat
1 large onion, sliced
½ green pepper, diced (optional)
1 8-oz. can tomato sauce
1 teaspoon salt
1 teaspoon Worcestershire sauce
6 hamburger buns

Melt bacon fat in a skillet; add loose meat, onion and pepper. Cook, stirring occasionally, until meat has lost its pink color. Add tomato sauce and seasonings. Continue to simmer about 5 minutes. Spoon into toasted hamburger buns.

CREOLE MEAT BALLS

(6 Family Servings)

Meat Balls

1 pound ground chuck
1 cup corn flake crumbs or fine dry bread crumbs
1 teaspoon salt
1 egg
¼ cup tomato juice

Sauce

1 cup (8-oz. can) tomato sauce
2 tablespoons molasses
½ cup minced celery
1 teaspoon instant minced onion
2 tablespoons minced green pepper
½ cup tomato juice
Juice of 1 lemon
Dash of Tabasco sauce

Form the meat balls by combining ground meat, crumbs, salt, egg and tomato juice; blend well, make into 12 balls. Combine sauce ingredients; heat in heavy saucepan or top-of-stove casserole to simmering; add meat balls to sauce, cover, turn heat low, cook 25 minutes. Remove cover once to stir. Serve over hot, cooked rice.

CHEESEBURGERS

Prepare hamburgers by either of preceding recipes. Before removing from skillet, place a slice of American cheese over each patty, turn off heat, cover skillet about 1 minute. There should be enough retained heat in the skillet to partially melt the cheese. Transfer to buns with a spatula or pancake turner.

BASIC-FOUR MEAT LOAF

(6 Family Servings)

This meat loaf contains some of all the Basic Four essentials in one well-balanced dish!

- ½ cup beef bouillon
- 2 slices white or cracked wheat bread
- 1 pound ground beef
- 2 tablespoons minced parsley
- ⅔ cup instant nonfat dry milk
- ½ cup grated carrot
- 1 teaspoon instant minced onion, reconstituted
- 1 teaspoon lemon juice
- 1 egg yolk
- 1 teaspoon salt
- Dash of pepper
- ¼ cup tomato catsup

Heat bouillon (from can or made with powdered stock concentrate) to boiling; pour over bread in a bowl, let bread soak until soft. In a larger mixing bowl, combine beef, milk, parsley, carrot and softened onion, lemon juice, egg, salt and pepper. Add the soaked bread, work into the meat mixture until well-blended. Place meat mixture in open roasting pan, shape with fingers into a loaf. Spread tomato catsup over top. Bake in oven preheated to 350°F for 50 minutes to 1 hour.

To make gravy with pan drippings: Remove meat loaf to platter, using a pancake turner. Pour off and discard all but 2 tablespoons of pan drippings; stir 2 tablespoons flour into reserved drippings, cook, stirring over low heat until mixture bubbles. Slowly add 1 cup water, stirring, until smooth and thickened. If you like a rich gravy, after heat has been turned off, add 2 tablespoons heavy cream or sour cream.

TOMATO-AND-CHIP BURGERS

Prepare hamburgers by either of preceding recipes. Serve in toasted buns topped with sliced tomatoes and 2 or 3 large potato chips. As the bun is closed, the potato chips will be crushed enough to be easy to eat and they add a pleasantly salty flavor to both tomatoes and burgers.

FRANKFURTER SPANISH RICE

(2 Child Servings)

- 2 tablespoons bacon fat or butter
- ¼ cup chopped onion
- 2 tablespoons chopped green pepper
- 2 frankfurters, thickly sliced
- ⅔ cup packaged precooked rice
- ¾ cup boiling hot water
- 1 8-oz. can tomato sauce
- ½ teaspoon salt
- 1 tablespoon minced parsley

Heat bacon fat in skillet; add onion, green pepper and frankfurters. Saute until lightly browned. Add remaining ingredients; mix well. Bring quickly to a boil, reduce heat and simmer uncovered for 5 minutes.

HAMBURGER SPAGHETTI SAUCE

(4 Servings)

- ½ pound hamburger meat
- 2 tablespoons olive oil
- 1 medium onion, chopped
- 1 garlic clove, minced
- 2 tablespoons minced fresh parsley
- 1 8-oz. can tomato sauce
- 1 1-lb. can whole peeled tomatoes
- ½ cup shredded American cheese

Saute meat in olive oil in a skillet until lightly browned, stirring with a fork. Add onion, garlic and parsley; cook over reduced heat until onion is soft. Add tomato sauce and peeled tomatoes; cook uncovered over reduced heat, breaking up peeled tomatoes with a fork. When sauce has cooked down and is thickened, about 30 minutes, add the cheese, stir until cheese is melted. Serve over hot cooked spaghetti.

MEAT BALLS AND SPAGHETTI

(6 Family Servings)

1 lb. hamburger meat or ground chuck
1 teaspoon salt
⅓ cup instant nonfat dry milk (optional)
1 egg
¼ cup crushed cracker crumbs
2 tablespoons very cold water
1 teaspoon shortening
2 cups spaghetti sauce
1 1-lb package thin spaghetti, cooked
Grated Parmesan cheese

Combine meat, salt, dry milk, egg and crumbs. Blend lightly with fingers, working in the cold water. Form into balls ¾ to 1 inch in diameter. Saute the meatballs in the shortening until well-browned on all sides. Add the spaghetti sauce (a prepared commercial sauce or a favorite homemade sauce). Simmer meat balls in the sauce, uncovered, for 15 to 20 minutes. Serve over hot cooked spaghetti; pass the grated Parmesan.

DANISH CHOPPED STEAK

(6 Family Servings)

1½ lbs. ground chuck or round beef
2 slices white or cracked wheat bread, soaked in ½ cup milk
1 egg
1 teaspoon salt
¼ teaspoon pepper
¼ cup seasoned flour
3 or 4 tablespoons bacon fat
2 large onions, sliced
4 tablespoons beef-flavored brown gravy mix
1½ cups water

Combine beef with the soaked bread, egg, salt and pepper. Work together until smooth. Form into 6 large plump meat patties. Dredge meat patties with seasoned flour. Heat bacon fat in a skillet; saute the meat patties until very brown and crisp on each side. Remove patties to a platter; keep warm. Fry onions in the pan drippings until slightly browned. With a slotted spoon, remove onions from pan, pile on over meat patties. Pour off all excess fat from pan, leaving only 2 tablespoons fat. Combine beef-flavored brown gravy mix and water, add to skillet, simmer until well-blended, smooth and thickened. Pour gravy over the meat patties and onions.

BARBECUED SPARERIBS

(6 to 8 Family Servings)

4 lbs. lean pork spareribs, cut in ribs
¼ cup brown sugar
1 tablespoon salt
1 tablespoon chili powder
½ cup catsup
1 or 2 garlic cloves, crushed
½ cup syrup from canned peaches
¼ cup vinegar
Dash of powdered cloves
½ cup water

Place ribs in a large shallow pan. Combine remaining ingredients in a saucepan, bring to a boil. Pour mixture over ribs and let stand several hours. To barbecue over charcoal, remove ribs from marinade, place on grid 5 inches from heat, baste the marinade over the meat as it cooks, turning frequently until ribs are well-browned, about 30 minutes. These are very spicy but even children who normally shy away from highly-seasoned foods seem to like them.

LONDON BROIL TETRAZZINI

(4 Family Servings)

1½ pounds top round, cut 1½ inches thick
Meat tenderizer
¼ cup soy sauce
¼ cup orange juice
Pinch of powdered ginger (optional)
2 tablespoons wine vinegar

Punch holes in the meat with a skewer, on both sides. Moisten with water, then sprinkle commercial meat tenderizer over the surface of meat, sprinkling generously. Let stand 5 minutes. Combine soy sauce, orange juice, ginger, and vinegar. Pour over meat. Let meat soak in mixture 30 minutes or longer. Broil 4 inches from heat for 10 minutes on each side for rare. Slice at an angle in very thin slices.

CHILI CON CARNE

(4 Servings)

½ lb. chopped beef (hamburger meat)
2 tablespoons oil
1 large onion, chopped
2 garlic cloves, minced
1 teaspoon chili powder, or more to taste
¼ teaspoon cumin (optional)
¼ teaspoon oregano
1 1-lb. can whole peeled tomatoes
1 1-lb. can red kidney beans, drained
1 teaspoon beef stock concentrate; or 1 beef bouillon cube
1 cup water
1 cup cooked rice

Saute the beef in oil until lightly browned; add onion and garlic, cook until soft. Stir in chili powder, cumin and oregano. Cook, stirring, until well-mixed. Add tomatoes, kidney beans, and beef stock concentrate or bouillon cube, and water. Simmer uncovered 20 to 30 minutes longer. Add rice, cook about 2 minutes.

BEEF KABOBS

(6 Family Servings)

1½ pounds beef chuck cut into cubes about 1½ inches
Meat tenderizer
½ cup olive oil
¼ cup vinegar
2 tablespoons orange juice
1 teaspoon salt

Place cubes of meat in large bowl. Sprinkle with water to moisten all sides, then sprinkle generously with commercial meat tenderizer. Let stand 5 minutes. Combine olive oil, vinegar, orange juice and salt; pour over meat, let stand in marinade at least 1 hour. Remove from marinade, put cubes of beef on skewers, broil over charcoal, turning frequently until well-browned on all sides.

(These can be broiled in the broiling oven or on a rotisserie spit, but they must be turned frequently.)

Chicken and Turkey

Fried chicken and roast turkey are two dishes which all children seem to adore. Since these are standard dishes in all American families, there seems no need to give recipes for them here. Most of the following are suggested ways to serve chicken parts to children on evenings when parents are out, or ways to make use of leftover chicken or turkey.

SOUTHERN FRIED CHICKEN

(4 Family Servings)

1 3-lb. chicken, cut up	1 teaspoon salt
2 cups buttermilk	½ teaspoon black pepper
1 cup flour	½ cup shortening

Marinate chicken pieces in buttermilk for 1 hour. Remove from buttermilk; dredge chicken pieces with flour which has been blended with salt and pepper. (Marinating the chicken in buttermilk makes it especially tender and of course provides additional nutrition.) Heat shortening in a large heavy skillet; fry chicken pieces until crisply browned on all sides. Remove with slotted spoon; drain on paper towel.

TURKEY HASH ON TOAST

This can be made with any little scraps of turkey left on the bones. Simply heat the chopped turkey in leftover gravy until the gravy bubbles, then spoon over buttered toast. (If there isn't enough leftover gravy, used canned chicken gravy.) Sprinkle a little minced parsley on top, or garnish with quartered hard-cooked eggs.

If the amount of turkey meat is skimpy, a little leftover bread stuffing can be added to the gravy as an extender.

CRISP OVEN-FRIED DRUMSTICKS

(4 Child Servings)

A good choice on nights when a baby-sitter is taking over. Drumsticks can be prepared in advance, slipped into oven to cook. Or, if oven can be clock-set to turn on and turn off at certain times, the drumsticks can be placed in oven before parents leave.

4 drumsticks
½ cup melted margarine
½ teaspoon salt
¾ to 1 cup corn flake crumbs

Wash drumsticks and pat dry with paper towel. Melt margarine in small skillet, stir in salt, dip drumsticks in the mixture. Roll drumsticks in the corn flake crumbs until well-coated. Place in shallow baking pan lined with aluminum foil. Bake in oven preheated to 350°F for one hour, turning once.

CHICKEN À LA KING

(4 family Servings)

2 cups diced cooked chicken meat, or leftover cooked turkey
2 tablespoons butter
2 tablespoons minced or finely sliced onion
½ green pepper, diced
1 canned pimiento, drained, diced
2 tablespoons flour
2 teaspoons chicken stock concentrate
1½ cups milk
1 tablespoon sherry (optional)

Melt butter in saucepan; add onion, green pepper and pimiento and cook over moderate heat until onion is soft. Stir in flour and chicken stock concentrate, then slowly add milk. Stir and cook until sauce is thickened and smooth. Add sherry and diced chicken (or turkey) and simmer 15 minutes. (*The alcohol in the sherry will evaporate, leaving only flavor.*) Serve with rice.

Optional addition: 2 hard-cooked eggs, quartered. Add these with the diced cooked chicken to extend number of servings.

BARBECUED CHICKEN WINGS

(4 Child Servings)

8 chicken wings
1 cup prepared barbecue sauce
½ cup orange juice
1 teaspoon Worcestershire sauce

Marinate chicken wings in the combined barbecue sauce, orange juice and Worcestershire for ½ to 1 hour. Arrange in foil-lined broiler pan. Broil 6 inches from heat, turning several times, until crisply browned—but take care that they do not burn (the sweetening in the barbecue sauce may cause them to char before being thoroughly cooked.) Twenty-five minutes should be ample cooking time.

CHICKEN AND DUMPLINGS

(4 Family Servings)

1 3-lb. chicken, cut up
1½ teaspoons salt, or 2 chicken bouillon cubes or 2 teaspoons chicken stock concentrate
1 cup biscuit mix
⅓ cup milk
1 egg
Minced parsley

Place chicken parts in Dutch oven, pressure cooker, or heavy kettle. Add water enough to reach almost to the top of the chicken pieces, but not covering chicken (about 3 cups water). Add salt or bouillon cubes or chicken stock concentrate. Cover tightly, cook until chicken is tender, about 30 minutes. (In a pressure cooker, this requires only 15 minutes at 15 pounds pressure.) Combine biscuit mix, milk and egg; beat just to blend. Spoon this dough over top of chicken, sprinkle parsley over the dumpling dough. Replace cover, cook over low heat (but not at pressure) for 12 minutes. In serving, spoon the chicken broth over both chicken pieces and dumplings.

QUICK CHICKEN TETRAZZINI

(3 to 4 Family Servings)

- ½ 8-oz. package spaghetti, cooked
- 1 to 2 cups * diced cooked chicken
- 1 can condensed cream of chicken soup
- ⅓ cup light cream
- 1 egg, beaten
- 1 3-oz. can mushrooms, well-drained (optional)
- ½ cup fine dry crumbs
- ½ cup grated Parmesan cheese
- 1 tablespoon butter

In a greased 1½-quart casserole, arrange spaghetti in layers with the chicken; combine soup, cream, egg, and drained mushrooms, spoon some of this mixture over each layer of chicken. Spread crumbs blended with cheese over top layer; dot with butter. Bake in oven preheated to 350°F for 50 minutes until sauce bubbles and crumbs are lightly browned.

* The more chicken, the better—but if you have only a little chicken available, the dish can still be prepared. Or, substitute cooked turkey for chicken in above recipe to make **Quick Turkey Tetrazzini.**

Fish and Seafood

Most American children rebel at fish, for the same reason as their elders: because so little genuinely fresh fish is available in most American markets. Children who have grown up in coastal communities or in households where fish dishes are popular with the family may not put up a fuss at all. But even if children do not like fish, it is very good for them—especially tuna, which contains important fish oil, a source of Vitamin D.

BAKED TUNA CHOW MEIN

(4 Child Servings)

2 cups (1 can) Chinese fried noodles
1 7-oz. can chunk style tuna, drained
1 tablespoon butter
¼ cup minced onions
1 cup minced celery
½ green pepper, diced
1 can condensed cream of mushroom soup
⅓ cup light cream or milk
1 teaspoon soy sauce

Arrange half the noodles in the bottom of a shallow baking dish, 9 x 9 x 2 inches. Flake tuna, spread over the noodles. Melt butter in saucepan, saute onions, celery and pepper until soft. Add soup, cream or milk, and soy sauce. Cook, stirring, until well-blended. Pour over tuna. Top with remaining noodles. Bake at 350°F for about 30 minutes.

FISH STICKS CREOLE

(4 Child Servings)

1 package frozen fish sticks
1 tablespoon butter or margarine
2 tablespoons minced onion
4 tablespoons minced celery
½ green pepper, minced; or ¼ cup sliced or chopped pimiento-stuffed olives
1 15-oz. jar spaghetti sauce (or 2 cups spaghetti sauce made with mix)
½ cup grated Parmesan cheese

Place fish sticks in shallow baking pan or dish, 9 x 9 x 2 inches. Bake in oven preheated to 400°F until fish sticks are crisply browned. Meantime, saute the onion, celery and green pepper (or olives) in butter; when onion is soft, add the spaghetti sauce and continue cooking over low heat about 10 minutes. Pour over fish sticks. Sprinkle cheese over sauce. Return to oven, bake 10 to 15 minutes longer. This is very good with baked potatoes (which can be placed in the oven to bake 1 hour before dinner is to be served, then, when it is time to place the fish sticks in the oven, it will already be heated to 400°F).

Short-cut Variation: Instead of sauteing onions, celery and green pepper in butter, simply add 1 teaspoon instant minced onion and 2 tablespoons minced celery to prepared spaghetti sauce with 1 tablespoon oil (preferably olive oil) and heat thoroughly. Add 1 teaspoon minced parsley to this sauce before pouring it over the fish sticks.

Meat Substitutes

TOMATO-CROWNED MACARONI AND CHEESE

Place slices of tomato over top of individual servings of frozen macaroni and cheese; dot tomato slices with butter and sprinkle minced parsley over top, then dribble with just a few drops of olive oil. Bake as usual according to package directions.

ITALIAN-STYLE BAKED MACARONI

(2 Servings)

1 cup elbow macaroni, cooked
1 8-oz. can tomato sauce
¼ teaspoon oregano
1 tablespoon instant minced onion
2 tablespoons minced fresh parsley
1 tablespoon olive oil
½ cup ricotta or cottage cheese
Sliced mozzarella or grated Parmesan cheese

Place half the cooked macaroni in the bottom of a greased 1-quart casserole. Combine tomato sauce, oregano, instant onion, parsley and olive oil; spread half this mixture over the macaroni. Spread the ricotta or cottage cheese over the tomato sauce. Add remaining macaroni and remaining sauce. Top with cheese. Bake in oven preheated to 350°F for a half-hour, until cheese is melted and sauce bubbling.

SPAGHETTI WITH TOMATO-CHEESE SAUCE

(4 to 6 Child Servings)

Stir 1 cup grated American cheese into 1 cup prepared spaghetti sauce or tomato sauce, stirring with a whisk until cheese is melted. Serve this over hot cooked spaghetti (½ of an 8-oz. package), sprinkling a little minced parsley over the top. Most younger children seem to prefer the flavor of American cheese to that of Parmesan.

EASY MACARONI AND CHEESE BAKE

(2 Servings)

- 1 cup elbow macaroni, cooked
- 1 cup diced or grated American cheese
- ½ cup commercial sour cream
- 2 tablespoons butter or margarine
- Salt, pepper

Place half of macaroni in bottom of greased 1-quart casserole. Add half the cheese and half the sour cream. Sprinkle with salt and pepper. Add remaining macaroni, cheese and sour cream and again sprinkle with salt and pepper. Bake covered in a 350°F oven for a half-hour.

PINEAPPLE BAKED BEANS

(2 to 3 Servings)

- 1 1-lb. can or jar New England style baked beans
- 1 teaspoon prepared mustard
- 2 tablespoons molasses
- 2 tablespoons tomato catsup or chili sauce
- 6 to 8 chunks (1-inch cubes) American cheese
- 4 canned pineapple slices

Empty beans into a 1-quart casserole. Stir into beans the mustard, catsup, and 1 tablespoon molasses. Push cheese down into the beans with a spoon. Over the top, arrange pineapple slices. Dribble a little molasses (about 1 tablespoonful) over top of pineapple. Bake uncovered in oven preheated to 400°F until sauce is bubbling and pineapple glazed to a light brown.

VEGE-TOMATO SAUCE FOR SPAGHETTI

(2 Cups)

1 small carrot, grated
1 small onion, minced
1 celery stick, minced
2 tablespoons minced parsley
¼ teaspoon dried thyme
¼ teaspoon oregano
2 tablespoons butter or margarine
1 1-lb. can peeled whole tomatoes
1 6-oz. can tomato paste
1 teaspoon sugar
Salt to taste
½ cup grated American cheese

Cook the carrots, onion, celery and parsley in butter over moderately low heat until very soft but not browned. Add thyme and oregano, cook a few minutes longer. Add the whole tomatoes, forcing through a sieve into the pan. Let cook 5 minutes; add tomato paste, sugar and salt. Simmer uncovered 25 to 30 minutes over lowest heat. Stir in cheese, beating with a whisk, until cheese is melted. (If a smoother sauce is preferred, after sauce is sufficiently cooked, beat in blender a moment, just before serving.)

Vegetables

It's been my experience that children who don't like vegetables to begin with are even less tempted when the vegetables are dressed up with sauces or special seasoning. Vegetables should be as briefly cooked as possible (some should still be slightly crisp), and in the smallest possible amount of water. In most cases, children will prefer them seasoned with nothing more than salt and butter (perhaps a dash of monosodium glutamate to bring out natural flavor).

The most valuable of all vegetables nutritionally are *carrots, green beans, tomatoes, broccoli, spinach, celery, greens* (mustard, turnip and beet greens) and the various members of the *cabbage family.*

Quick tips for preparing these vegetables, to retain maximum flavor, color and food value, are suggested.

ASPARAGUS

Scrub spears with vegetable brush to rid them of sand. Break off tough stem ends. Place spears horizontally in a skillet with water barely to cover; add salt. Place lid over skillet so that it covers most of the pan but allows escape of steam. (Steam dulls the bright color.) Cook just until spears can be pierced with a fork, about 6 minutes. Drain off part but not all of the cooking liquid; add a lump of butter or margarine. Serve this way or on toast (sprinkle some of the cooking liquid over the toast as a sauce).

BEETS AND BEET GREENS

The leaves of the beets are very rich in Vitamin A and a better source of potassium and iron than the beet roots. It's a good idea to dish them up together. First, parboil the beet *roots* without peeling. Allow them to cool, then rub off the skins. Slice or chop the beets.

Meantime, select the best of the beet tops (discard those that are brownish or badly wilted), soak in a sinkful of water to get rid of all dirt or grit. Drain well; place in a pot with just a little water and a sprinkling of salt. Simmer tightly covered for about 10 minutes; drain well. Place in pan with sliced or chopped beetroot, with margarine or oil and a dash of vinegar (2 tablespoons of margarine or oil, 1 teaspoon vinegar for 2 cups beet greens before cooking). A little dry mustard also may be added, if desired. The slightly bitter flavor of the greens is pleasantly offset by the sweetness of the beetroot.

BROCCOLI

An excellent source of calcium, phosphorus, and Vitamin A. Separate the flowerlets, cut off tough portion of stems, and place in already-boiling salted water, partially covered (so steam can escape). Cook just until flowerlets can be pierced with a fork, about 10 minutes. Serve dressed with butter or margarine, or with oil and lemon juice.

BRUSSELS SPROUTS

Trim sprouts, cook as described for broccoli, but only about 5 minutes, just until largest can be pierced with fork. These have infinitely better flavor when cooked until barely tender, still bright green in color. Dress with butter. (Leftover cooked sprouts are good dressed with olive oil and vinegar, served cold as a salad.)

CABBAGE

Your children will probably prefer this in the form of cole slaw, but when it is served cooked, turn off the heat as soon as the cabbage is fork-tender but still slightly crisp and has not turned pale. Very good dressed with sour cream and poppy seeds or toasted sesame seeds, or with sauteed almonds or pine nuts.

CARROTS

If cut fine enough, these can be cooked in butter only—no liquid, and 5 minutes' cooking time is enough. Either slice them horizontally or cut lengthwise in "sticks." Sometimes I precook them in a very small amount of water for 2 minutes, drain the water, then add butter and cook tightly covered another 2 or 3 minutes. A little minced parsley or minced fresh dill adding just before serving makes them more attractive in both appearance and flavor.

GLAZED CARROTS

A French cooking trick, well worth knowing about. Cut carrots lengthwise in quarters. Cook in 1 cup seasoned chicken broth (you may use 1 teaspoon chicken stock concentrate and 1 cup water). Cook uncovered at moderately high heat until liquid cooks down to one-third. Add 1 teaspoon sugar and 1 tablespoon butter, continue cooking until liquid is thickened and glazed.

CELERY

Popular as celery is when eaten raw, it is equally good cooked and served as a vegetable, in any one of the three ways which follow.

CELERY IN BUTTER SAUCE

(4 Family Servings)

4 large sticks celery, sliced at an angle
2 tablespoons butter
½ cup water
½ teaspoon salt

Place celery, butter, water and salt in saucepan. Cook, tightly covered, about 12 minutes or until tender. Uncover, reduce liquid over high heat. Remove celery with slotted spoon. (Save any remaining liquid for use in sauces or gravies.)

Celery in Chicken Broth: Use 1 teaspoon chicken stock concentrate instead of salt.

CELERY AND TOMATOES

(4 Family Servings)

1 small onion, thinly sliced
1 medium tomato, chopped
2 tablespoons butter
4 large celery stalks, sliced at an angle
¼ teaspoon salt

Saute onion and tomato in butter until onion is yellow and soft. Add celery and salt, cook, covered, until celery is quite tender, about 15 minutes. Serve this way with cooking liquid as a sauce.

COLLARD, MUSTARD GREENS, TURNIP GREENS, KALE, ETC.

All these greens are cooked in the same way. First soak in water to remove all grit or sand; drain well, then place in a large kettle with a small amount of water, about ½ cup, and sprinkle with salt from a shaker. Cook tightly covered for approximately 10 minutes or until leaves are very soft. Drain. Dress with butter or margarine, or with oil and a dash of vinegar, or with crumbled cooked bacon and bacon fat. All greens are prime sources of Vitamin C, even when cooked, and rich in important minerals.

GREEN BEANS

You're always safe with these, probably the most popular of all vegetables with children (and most adults, too). Easiest way is to break beans into 1-inch lengths, though cooking time is slightly shorter if slit lengthwise. Cooking time in boiling salted water is 8 to 10 minutes. Frozen beans have same food value, but less flavor. Beans need no other seasoning than a lump of butter.

PEAS

Frozen peas can be very delicious if cooked only in butter, no liquid—or use 2 tablespoons each butter and water. Another way is to saute just a little onion in butter first, then add the block of frozen peas and cook until peas have defrosted enough to break up the frozen block. Cover peas with lettuce leaves (preferably Boston lettuce), cover the saucepan tightly, and cook over low heat about 5 minutes. Discard lettuce before serving.

Fresh peas, shelled, require about 15 minutes cooking in boiling salted water, but less water is needed if shelled peas are covered by lettuce leaves during cooking.

SPINACH

To retain its full flavor, spinach should not be cooked more than 3 or 4 minutes—just until wilted. Trim off the stems and soak the leaves well, in a large quantity of water, then remove the well-soaked leaves to a kettle and sprinkle lightly with salt. *Do not add additional water.* The moisture clinging to the leaves is enough. Bring to a boil, tightly covered; lower heat. After 3 minutes, check to see if leaves are wilted. Drain immediately, pushing out the water or chopping leaves with a knife to force water out. Add a lump of butter. Or squeeze fresh lemon juice over spinach to taste. In our house, this has always been a favorite vegetable. An excellent source of Vitamin A, calcium and phosphorus.

SWEET POTATOES

A great source of Vitamin A and nearly all children like them —especially when candied. The canned candied Louisiana yams have the same food value as freshly cooked yams, though they are not quite as flavorful (what canned vegetables are?). Baked sweet potatoes (or yams) are very easy: simply stick them in the oven, as you do to bake white potatoes, cut open the skins when they are fork-tender and add a lump of butter to each potato.

SWISS CHARD

This looks like a salad green, with large green leaves and white stems, but it's a little too bitter to serve raw. Cook like other greens in a small amount of water with salt, drain well, serve hot, dressed with oil and vinegar. Excellent for Vitamin A and calcium.

TOMATOES

A few children here and there are allergic to tomatoes, but are less bothered by thoroughly cooked tomatoes (as when baked or in sauce) than the raw. A top source of Vitamin C, even after cooking and canning.

ESCALLOPED TOMATOES

(4 Family Servings)

1 large can (1 lb., 12 oz.) tomatoes
½ teaspoon salt
1 teaspoon sugar
¼ teaspoon oregano (optional)
¼ teaspoon thyme (optional)
2 slices stale white bread, in cubes
2 tablespoons butter

Empty tomatoes into baking dish 10 x 10 x 2 inches (do not use metal pan). Add salt, sugar, and herbs (if desired), stir to distribute through tomatoes. Push bread down into the tomatoes so that it is completely covered. Dot butter over the top. Bake at 400°F for 1 to 1½ hours, or at 350°F for 2 to 2½ hours (easy with an oven meal, to accompany a roast).

ITALIAN-STYLE FRIED TOMATOES

(4 Family Servings)

3 to 4 tablespoons butter
2 large tomatoes, thickly sliced
¼ teaspoon oregano
¼ teaspoon thyme
Salt, pepper

Melt butter in a large skillet over low heat. Add tomatoes; sprinkle with herbs, salt and pepper. Cook slowly until lightly browned on bottom; turn carefully with spatula or pancake turner and cook until golden on the other side. Keep heat low at all times. Excellent with scrambled eggs for brunch or week-end breakfasts.

WHITE POTATOES

These are a very good source of phosphorus and potassium and contain no more calories per serving than green peas or lima beans. Children usually prefer them mashed or French fried, and will settle for packaged mashed potatoes and frozen French fries without complaint (which is a help for those parents who are skipping starch foods for dietary reasons).

The following recipe is given because it is quick and easy and a change from the sogginess of frozen French fries.

COTTAGE-FRIED POTATOES

Peel potatoes, slice crosswise as thin as possible. Saute in melted bacon fat or vegetable shortening in a covered skillet until well-browned and fork-tender, turning with a pancake turner once or twice, replacing cover after each turning. Requires about 15 minutes cooking time.

Salads, Raw Vegetables, Relishes

For the most part, children prefer their roughage in finger form. Cole slaw, potato salad, and molded vegetable or vegetable and fruit salads are the exceptions. Since vegetables in the raw state are a better source of Vitamin C than when cooked, you are quite justified in pampering this whim. Keep carrot sticks, trimmed celery sticks, and cucumbers (if these are popular), ready to eat in plastic bags in the refrigerator. On occasion, green beans, if young and tender, are also preferred raw.

CARROT COLE SLAW

(4 to 6 Family Servings)

2 cups shredded cabbage
2 large carrots, scraped, grated
1 teaspoon minced scallion (optional)
½ teaspoon salt, or to taste
¼ cup mayonnaise
¼ cup commercial sour cream
½ teaspoon sugar
1 teaspoon vinegar
½ teaspoon poppy seeds or caraway seeds (optional)

Combine cabbage, carrot and minced scallion in bowl. Sprinkle with salt, stir to blend well. Add remaining ingredients, toss well. Serve cold garnished with green pepper strips and slices of hard-cooked egg.

PINEAPPLE COLE SLAW

(4 to 6 Family Servings)

3 cups shredded cabbage
½ green pepper, diced
½ cup crushed pineapple
½ teaspoon salt or to taste
Freshly ground black pepper
1 teaspoon vinegar
½ cup Boiled Dressing (see below)
Paprika

Combine cabbage, green pepper and pineapple. Season with salt and pepper. Stir in vinegar and the Boiled Dressing; blend well. Sprinkle paprika over top before serving.

WILTED LETTUCE

(4 Family Servings)

3 slices bacon
4 to 6 cups garden or Boston lettuce, torn in large pieces
⅓ cup vinegar
2 tablespoons sugar

Cook bacon until crisp; remove, drain bacon on paper towel. Add lettuce to the hot bacon fat in skillet, cover, let stand 5 minutes. Add vinegar and sugar and the crumbled cooked bacon. Toss to blend. Serve as a vegetable.

(*Note:* Spinach can also be prepared the same way.)

BOILED DRESSING

(Makes 2 Cups)

1½ teaspoons salt
1 teaspoon prepared mustard
1½ tablespoons sugar
½ tablespoon flour
2 egg yolks
1½ tablespoons butter, melted
¾ cup milk
¼ cup vinegar

Combine salt, mustard, sugar and flour, blend well. Beat in egg yolks, then melted butter. Place over hot water in top of double boiler, slowly add milk, then vinegar, stirring constantly with a whisk until sauce thickens. Or, if you have an electric blender, put all ingredients in blender at once (butter need not be melted) and beat until smooth, then transfer to saucepan over lowest heat, stirring constantly with whisk until mixture thickens and is smooth and creamy. Very good both on cole slaw and potato salad. Children like its sweet-sour tang.

COTTAGE CHEESE TOMATO SALAD

(4 Family Servings)

1 cup cottage cheese
2 gherkin pickles, chopped
1 small carrot grated
1 teaspoon grated onion
Salt, pepper
4 medium tomatoes
Mayonnaise or Thousand Island Dressing

Combine cottage cheese, pickles, carrot, onion and salt and pepper. Stir in about 2 tablespoons mayonnaise or Thousand Island Dressing. Cut tomatoes partway through in quarters so that they spread out like flower petals. Sprinkle salt over tomatoes, then top each with cottage cheese mixture. Top each serving with a spoonful of dressing.

BEAN SALAD

(4 Servings)

1 cup cooked or canned green beans
1 cup cooked lima beans
1 hard-cooked egg, chopped
4 or 5 black olives, chopped
3 tablespoons oil
½ teaspoon salt
1 tablespoon vinegar
Pinch of sugar
4 cups (approx.) salad greens

Combine beans, chopped egg, chopped olives, oil, salt, vinegar and sugar. Blend well; marinate until time to serve. Add salad greens, toss. (If children do not want the salad greens, select the beans and egg from the bowl—these are more important nutritionally than the lettuce.)

CREAM DRESSING FOR LETTUCE SALAD

(Makes ¾ Cup)

½ cup light cream
1 teaspoon sugar
¼ cup vinegar
¼ teaspoon salt

Combine ingredients, pour over shredded or torn lettuce. Enough for 4 to 6 servings.

CANADIAN APPLE SALAD

(6 to 8 Family Servings)

This makes a fine wintertime salad.

2 large tart apples, chopped
2 sticks green celery, chopped
6 walnut halves, chopped
1 raw white turnip, peeled, cut in slivers
1 tablespoon green pepper, chopped
8 pitted dates, chopped
Shredded Swiss cheese, about ¼ cup
French dressing, or mayonnaise
Iceberg lettuce, in cups

This can be served either on individual salad plates or served from a salad bowl. If preparing individual servings, combine all ingredients but cheese, dressing and lettuce; blend and spoon mixture onto a lettuce cup in each plate. Top with a spoonful of cheese and pass dressing or mayonnaise to be taken to individual taste. If preparing salad in a bowl, combine all ingredients except lettuce; toss to blend, serve over lettuce.

GOLDEN GLOW SALAD

(6 Servings)

1 3-oz. package lemon-flavored gelatin
½ teaspoon salt
1½ cups hot water
⅔ cup drained crushed pineapple
⅓ cup pineapple juice
1 tablespoon lemon juice
1 cup grated raw carrot

Dissolve gelatin and salt in hot water. Add pineapple and juice and the lemon juice. Chill until gelatin is syrupy. Fold in the carrots. Pour into pan 9 x 9 x 2 inches. Chill until very firm, about 3 hours. Unmold by dipping pan in hot water, then invert. Cut into squares. Serve on crisp lettuce topped with mayonnaise.

Desserts

Pies and cakes are never hard to sell to children, even the finicky ones. The desserts suggested here have been chosen primarily for their nutritive value, so that when the finicky eaters are short on main course portions and long on desserts, they at least will be getting some of the food value they need.

STRAWBERRIES IN ORANGE JUICE

Simple, but so very good. Trim and wash strawberries, sugar them in the usual way and spoon into serving dishes. Over each serving, pour orange juice enough to cover berries. This gives the berries quite different flavor, a delicious change.

PEACHES IN MOCK CHAMPAGNE CUP

Peel fresh peaches, slice or cut in halves. Marinate in a mixture of half orange juice, half ginger ale.

AMBROSIA

Simple but delicious: peel, dice, and sugar oranges, top with shredded coconut. What a wonderful flavor lift the coconut gives! (Sometimes diced oranges are combined half and half with sliced bananas—also mighty good, and slightly less costly.)

PEACHES AND CREAM

Throughout the year, this makes a quick, easy and healthful dessert: serve canned peach halves topped with either light or heavy cream. Delicious plain, or use as a topping for slices of pound cake or squares of gingerbread.

ORANGE-NUT COMPOTE

Peel and dice oranges as for Ambrosia, but instead of coconut, add chopped walnuts. Sliced bananas may also be added, or halved seedless grapes, or fresh or canned peaches.

PEACH PUDDING

When making vanilla pudding with pudding and pie filling mix, use canned peach syrup in place of part of the milk; after pudding has thickened, stir in sliced canned peaches. Serve topped with whipped cream.

PINEAPPLE LEMON PUDDING

Prepare lemon pudding and pie filling mix according to package directions, but use ½ cup syrup from canned pineapple in place of same amount of water; after pudding has thickened, stir in ½ cup slivered pineapple chunks. Chill. Serve topped with whipped cream and slivered toasted almonds.

BANANA CHOCOLATE SUNDAE

Arrange sliced bananas atop each serving of vanilla ice cream, pour chocolate sauce over all, garnish with chopped nuts. Peanuts are good with this one.

BANANA SPLIT

Spoon vanilla ice cream into serving dishes; arrange banana halves, split lengthwise, over top. Sprinkle chopped walnuts over bananas and garnish with whipped cream and maraschino cherries. Always a winner.

BAKED PEACH CUSTARD

(6 Family Servings)

4 cups milk
4 eggs, beaten
½ cup sugar
Pinch of salt
2 fresh peaches, sliced, sugared
Nutmeg

Combine milk, eggs, sugar and salt; beat until foamy. Pour into Pyrex baking dish 10 x 10 x 2 inches, or into 6 individual Pyrex custard cups. Put 2 peach slices in each cup, or distribute peach slices in the single large custard. Sprinkle nutmeg over top. Set baking dish or custard cups in roasting pan, add warm water to depth of ½ inch. Bake in 350°F oven for 1 hour or until table knife inserted in center comes out clean.

LEMON SAUCE

(About 1¼ Cups)

1 lemon
2 egg yolks
1 cup water
2 tablespoons cornstarch
½ to ¾ cup sugar (according to degree of sweetness desired)
Pinch of salt

Peel lemon, removing only the thinnest part of the outer rind (none of the white membrane). Cut the peel in pieces and place in electric blender. Peel off white membrane from lemon, cut lemon in thin slices, removing seeds. Place seeded lemon slices in blender. Add egg yolks and water. Blend sugar and cornstarch, add this to blender. Beat at low speed until lemon is chopped and mixture well-blended; transfer to saucepan and cook, stirring constantly with a whisk over low heat, until thickened and creamy (lemon pieces will still form small lumps). Keep warm over hot water until needed. Leftover sauce may be refrigerated and reheated when needed. Very good over cake or puddings.

PINEAPPLE ANGEL SAUCE

(Makes 1 Cup)

2 egg yolks
⅓ cup frozen pineapple juice concentrate right from can
⅓ cup milk
½ cup sugar
⅓ cup softened butter

This is easy in a blender. Simply put all ingredients in the blender at once, beat until smooth, about 30 seconds. Pour into saucepan and cook, stirring constantly, over low heat until the sauce coats the spoon. Cool at room temperature. Serve over slices of angel food cake.

GRAPENUTS BROWN BETTY

(6 Servings)

3 large tart apples
¾ cup Grapenuts breakfast cereal
2 tablespoons brown sugar or molasses
½ teaspoon cinnamon
Pinch of salt
1 teaspoon grated lemon peel
1 tablespoon butter
Juice of ½ lemon

Peel and slice apples. Combine Grapenuts, sugar or molasses, cinnamon, salt, and grated lemon peel. Arrange alternate layers of Grapenuts mixture and apples in a 1½-quart baking dish, sprinkling lemon juice over the apple layers and dotting the Grapenuts layers with butter. Bake uncovered in oven preheated to 350°F for 30 minutes. Serve warm with Lemon Sauce (see recipe), heavy cream, or ice cream.

ORANGE CAKE SAUCE

(Makes 1 Cup)

¼ cup softened butter
¼ cup frozen orange juice concentrate right from can
¼ cup evaporated milk
½ cup brown sugar

Put all ingredients in electric blender, beat until smooth. Serve over cake, ice cream, or thin pancakes.

PEACH COBBLER

(6 Servings)

1 large can peach halves in syrup
1 tablespoon butter
1 cup biscuit mix
1 tablespoon sugar
⅓ cup heavy cream

Place drained peach halves in bottom of 1½-quart baking dish. Spoon half the peach syrup over them. Dot with butter. Combine biscuit mix with sugar and cream; stir with fork until well-blended, spoon mixture over top of peaches, spreading to cover. Bake in oven preheated to 375°F until crust is golden, about 20 minutes. Serve warm topped with hot Lemon Sauce (see recipe), or with cream.

JELLIED AMBROSIA

(6 to 8 Servings)

2 oranges, peeled and diced; or 1 can Mandarin oranges, drained
1 banana, sliced
½ cup seedless white grapes, halved
½ cup shredded coconut
1 3-oz. package lemon- or orange-flavored gelatin
1 cup hot water
12 ice cubes
½ cup heavy cream, whipped and sweetened

Prepare fruit, mix with coconut. Dissolve gelatin in hot water; add ice cubes, stir until most of ice has melted and gelatin started to set, then remove remaining ice with slotted spoon and discard. Add fruit and coconut mixture to the gelatin; transfer to 1½-quart gelatin mold or to a serving dish or 8- or 9-inch square baking pan. Chill until firm. Unmold and garnish with whipped cream. Or serve directly from serving dish, passing whipped cream individually.

FRUIT SALAD IN GELATIN

Encourage children to make this themselves: it's easy and quick. Simply drain a large-sized can of fruit salad in a sieve propped over a mixing bowl. While fruit is draining, dissolve a package of fruit-flavored gelatin (any favorite flavor) in hot water, as directed on package. Instead of the cold water called for, add 8 to 12 ice cubes, stir until cubes are mostly melted and gelatin has begun to thicken. Remove remaining bits of ice with slotted spoon. Add the drained fruit, stir to distribute in gelatin, then pour into a serving dish or individual Pyrex cups and chill until firm.

RASPBERRIES IN GELATIN

(6 Servings)

1 3-oz. package raspberry- or black cherry-flavored gelatin
1¼ cups hot water
1 package frozen raspberries
1 teaspoon lemon juice (optional)
½ cup miniature marshmallows
Whipped cream

Place gelatin in bowl, add hot water, stir to dissolve. Add lemon juice and the solidly frozen raspberries. Stir gently until fruit has completely separated and gelatin starts to set. Stir in marshmallows. Pour into 1-quart mold or into 6 individual ¾-cup molds or custard cups. Chill until firm. Serve topped with whipped cream.

JELLIED PEACHES

(6 Servings)

6 canned peach halves, well-drained
1 3-oz. package lemon- or orange-flavored gelatin
1¼ cups hot water
¾ cup canned peach syrup
1 teaspoon lemon juice

Place a peach half in each of 6 Pyrex custard cups or individual gelatin molds. Dissolve the gelatin in hot water; add peach syrup and lemon juice. Pour gelatin over peaches and chill until firm. Serve in the Pyrex cups topped with whipped cream; or unmold and serve on lettuce as a salad, topped with cottage cheese and mayonnaise.

COTTAGE CHEESE PIE

(6 to 8 Servings)

- 1 unbaked pie shell (9 inches)
- 1 egg white, unbeaten
- 2 whole eggs
- 1 egg yolk
- ½ cup sugar
- Pinch of salt
- ½ cup heavy cream
- 1 pound cottage cheese or ricotta
- 2 tablespoons flour
- 1 teaspoon grated lemon peel

Brush bottom of unbaked pie shell with the egg white; chill ½ hour. Using a blender or mixer, beat together the whole eggs and egg yolk, sugar, salt, cream and cottage cheese and flour until very smooth. Add grated lemon peel towards the end. Pour mixture into chilled pie shell. Preheat oven to 350°F and bake pie for 40 minutes or until table knife inserted in center comes out clean. Cool before serving.

Cookies

LACY OATMEAL COOKIES

(4 to 5 dozen)

- ¾ cup vegetable shortening
- 1 cup brown sugar, well-packed
- ½ cup granulated sugar
- 1 egg
- ¼ cup water
- 1 teaspoon vanilla extract
- 1 cup sifted all-purpose unbleached flour
- 1 teaspoon salt
- ½ teaspoon soda
- 3 cups oatmeal
- ½ cup raisins or nuts, chopped

Place shortening, sugars, egg, water and vanilla in mixing bowl; beat thoroughly. Sift together flour, salt and soda. Add to first mixture, beat to blend. Stir in oatmeal and raisins or nuts. Drop by teaspoonful on greased baking sheet. Bake in oven preheated to 350°F for 12 to 15 minutes, until delicately browned. Remove from baking sheet with spatula, cool on flat surface.

EASY COCONUT MACAROONS

(2 Dozen)

- 2⅔ cups flaked coconut
- ¾ cup sweetened condensed milk
- 1 egg, beaten
- ¼ teaspoon almond extract

Combine ingredients in a bowl, stir until well-mixed. Let stand 2 or 3 minutes. Preheat oven to 325°F. Spread brown paper on baking sheet, grease the paper. Drop mixture by teaspoonfuls on the brown paper, flatten with back of spoon. Bake for 25 minutes or until delicately golden. Remove immediately from baking sheet with spatula and cool on flat surface.

NO-BAKE PEANUT BUTTER BALLS

(About 2½ Dozen)

- 1¼ cups graham cracker crumbs (about 15 crackers)
- ¼ cup sugar
- ½ teaspoon cinnamon
- ½ teaspoon nutmeg
- ½ cup peanut butter (creamy or chunk style)
- ⅓ cup light corn syrup
- Confectioners' sugar

Combine crumbs, sugar, cinnamon and nutmeg; blend well. Add peanut butter and syrup, stir with spoon until dough is formed. With moistened hands, roll into ½-inch balls. Chill on waxed paper. When firm, roll in sifted confectioners' sugar.

BUTTER COOKIES

(About 5 Dozen)

½ pound butter
1 teaspoon vanilla
1½ cups sifted confectioners' sugar
1 egg
2 cups sifted all-purpose flour
4 teaspoons baking powder
¼ teaspoon salt
⅔ cup instant nonfat dry milk

Cream butter with vanilla in bowl of electric mixer. Gradually add confectioners sugar with mixer in motion until batter is fluffy. Add egg, beat until smooth. Sift together flour, baking powder and salt; add this gradually to creamed mixture, and finally add the nonfat dry milk. When dough is smooth, transfer to waxed paper and form into a roll 2 inches in diameter. Chill until firm. Cut in thin slices with long sharp knife and place on ungreased baking sheet. Sprinkle tops of cookies with coconut, nuts, or colored sugar sprinkles. Bake in oven preheated to 400°F until lightly browned, about 8 minutes. Remove from pan while warm.

Cut-out cookies: After chilling, dough may be rolled out on lightly floured board and cut into shapes with cookies cutter, if preferred. This is always fun for younger children, who love cutting out cookies, especially with cutters in animal shapes.

RAISIN CORNFLAKE COOKIES

(About 3 Dozen)

2 eggs
⅓ cup sugar
1⅔ cups cornflake crumbs
⅔ cup finely chopped walnuts
⅔ cup raisins
Pinch of salt
½ teaspoon vanilla

Grease a baking sheet. Beat eggs until foamy. Stir in sugar. Fold in cornflake crumbs, nuts, raisins, salt and vanilla. Stir until well-blended. Let mixture stand for 30 minutes. Meantime, preheat oven to 350°F. When mixture has been standing for 30 minutes, drop by teaspoonfuls onto greased baking sheet; bake 10 minutes or until delicately browned. While still warm, remove the cookies from the pan with a spatula. Cool before eating.

INDEX